The Catheter Introducers

Leslie A. Geddes and
LaNelle E. Geddes

contributing editors

Michael Boo

Bob Drake

Susan Yoder

Mobium Press, Chicago, IL 60610
1993

Mobium Press, Chicago, IL 60610

© 1993 by Cook Group Incorporated. All rights reserved
Published 1993
Printed in the United States of America

Library of Congress Catalog Card Number: 92-063032

ISBN 0-916371-13-1

Foreword

Several years ago, I urged Dr. Les Geddes to write a history of early angiographic and interventional pioneers. Little did I realize that when the book was complete, many of the pioneering physicians and researchers would be gone—Dotter, Sones, Judkins, and Gruentzig.

Sadly, only portions of their lives and works are documented by their own writing. Much of the information about them in this book came from the recollections of friends, spouses, and colleagues closely associated with them.

As I read the drafts of this book, I sometimes said to myself, "Is this so?" and answered, "Probably not entirely." It is important for all of us to remember that there were many contributors to angiography and interventional medicine. With time, facts meld into a consensus about who achieved what, and so only a few receive credit and recognition for their contributions. In the end, who invented what is really less important than the knowledge that medicine was changed forever by a few recognized leaders and thousands of unheralded contributors.

After reading the work of Les and LaNelle Geddes, I thank them for a job well done. They reported well on what they heard and read.

To those of you who remember and were a part of this exciting era, we salute you and we thank you.

Bill Cook
President
Cook Group Incorporated

Table of Contents

   6   Preface

   8   Chapter 1
Essentials *The Essentials of Diagnostic Angiography and Interventional Radiology*

22   Chapter 2
Sven Ivar Seldinger *Charting a New Course*

30   Chapter 3
Erik Boijsen *Educator and Inventor*

36   Chapter 4
Mason Sones *Inventing Tapered, Flexible-Tip Catheters*

44   Chapter 5
Melvin P. Judkins *Approaching the Heart from a Different Angle*

52   Chapter 6
Charles T. Dotter *Taking Catheters into Intervention*

70 Chapter 7
Andreas Gruentzig *Balloons from Switzerland*

78 Chapter 8
Kurt Amplatz *Innovation in Devices and Procedures*

90 Chapter 9
Cesare Gianturco *The Giant of Coils, Filters, and Stents*

102 Chapter 10
Sidney Wallace *Applying Interventional Radiology to Cancer Treatment*

112 Chapter 11
Constantin Cope *Pioneering Contributions to Diagnostic Techniques*

122 Time Line

134 Notes on Contributors

136 Illustration References

138 References

145 Index

Preface

In 1985, the same year that we began to research this book, four catheterization pioneers died: Judkins on January 28, Dotter on February 16, Sones on August 29, and Gruentzig on October 27. The first two died before the start of this project; the other two died after the start, but before personal interviews could be conducted. However, their surviving colleagues and spouses were able to provide a wealth of firsthand information, some of it by mail and the remainder through personal interviews.

The starting point in compiling the information for this book was an interview with Erik Boijsen, Judkins' mentor and mentor to countless other angiographers. Boijsen was attending a meeting in Chicago in April 1985, where we were fortunate to meet with him. From this meeting, we gained a greater perspective on the field of angiography and learned much about his and Judkins' development of the hook-tail catheter. Boijsen also supplied personal information about Judkins and was able to provide Seldinger's address.

We then visited Sweden in the summer of 1986 to interview Seldinger, who generously shared information about his discovery of the percutaneous entry technique.

E.K. Shirey, W.C. Sheldon, Beverly Cohn of the Cleveland Clinic, and Geraldine Sones provided considerable information about Mason Sones. Enid Ruble contributed a wealth of material on Charles Dotter. Eileen Judkins furnished information about her late husband's development of the selective coronary artery catheter. We obtained biographical information on Gruentzig from Maria Schlumpf, his colleague in Zurich, and from his associates at Emory University, especially Linda Greene and Spencer B. King III.

The chapters on Sven Seldinger, Erik Boijsen, Kurt Amplatz, Cesare Gianturco, Constantin Cope, and Sidney Wallace were made possible through personal interviews.

Seeking Inspiration
Purely scientific publications rarely devote space to recounting how an inspiration occurred, nor do they describe the sometimes arduous process involved in seeking inspiration. Too often important

personal points are omitted. The reader doesn't learn, for example, what personal motivations were involved. The many inevitable failures inventors encounter on the road to success and the general lack of initial acceptance of new ideas within the medical community are quickly glossed over.

This book is different. We wanted to provide the reader with interesting background material related to the formulation of new concepts and the subsequent development of new techniques. Each chapter discusses the major accomplishments and contributions of individual pioneers that led to the emergence of modern technologies. In addition, extensive historical information on catheterization is provided to demonstrate the continual progression of science.

The critical event that underlies modern interventional radiology is, first and foremost, the discovery of x-rays in 1895 by Roentgen, who used his technique to "see" bones. Soon after that development, research scientists introduced the use of contrast medium to visualize the vascular system. Although motion pictures were applied to radiology in the early days, the introduction of the image intensifier made it possible to obtain fluoroscopic information necessary for diagnosis and intervention.

The more recent addition of videotaping has allowed radiologists to create a permanent record that can be evaluated immediately and then viewed as often as desired to obtain the maximum amount of helpful information. The power injector has made it possible to obtain better images of rapidly changing circulation phases and consequently has stimulated the development of selective angiography.

Seldinger's discovery of the percutaneous entry technique in 1953 eliminated the need to perform a cut-down procedure to expose a vessel. The development of curved catheters by many physicians permitted safe, selective angiography. Creation of the balloon-tipped catheter, first by urologists, made pulmonary circulation easy to observe, leading to routine measurement of cardiac output by the thermal dilution method. Finally, the introduction of balloon catheters to dilate stenosed vessels brought interventional radiology to the hands of physicians around the world.

Thanks to Many

The authors are indebted to so many who patiently answered questions and provided pictures, reprints, and numerous helpful suggestions. Among these are Rudy Davis and John Hart of United States Catheter and Instrument Corporation, Glens Falls, New York; Ralph Lach of Mt. Carmel Hospital, Dayton, Ohio; Robert C. Stevens, formerly with Cordis Corporation, Miami; John Abele of Boston Scientific Corporation, Boston; P.K. Billimoria, a colleague of both Dotter and Judkins; Bill Cook and Ross Jennings of Cook Incorporated, Bloomington, Indiana; Cesare Gianturco, of the Carle Clinic, Urbana, Illinois; and Kurt Amplatz, of the University of Minnesota.

Leslie A. Geddes   LaNelle E. Geddes

All great discoveries are made by men whose feelings run ahead of their thinking.

C.H. Parkhurst

Ready, Fire, Aim!

Unknown

CHAPTER 1

The Essentials of Diagnostic Angiography and Interventional Radiology

Today, we take interventional radiology for granted, as if it has always been available. In 1895, when Roentgen published his paper, "On a New Kind of Rays," the field of interventional radiology was beyond the imagination of most human beings. Much has transpired since Roentgen's discovery to bring us to the point where diagnostic and interventional radiology now work hand in hand.

The interventional radiologist needs relatively few yet immeasurably important tools, including syringes and hypodermic needles, wire guides and catheters, and x ray images enhanced by contrast media. Each of these has undergone a long and circuitous route to reach its present-day configuration, beginning with the very thought of diagnosis.

Three major events paved the way to modern intervention: Forssmann's leap of faith in 1929, Seldinger's discovery of the percutaneous entry technique in 1953, and Dotter's first percutaneous arterial dilation in 1964. In addition, hundreds of lesser-known events have gradually shaped the tools and techniques of the interventional radiologist.

No single person perfected the common techniques that we recognize today. History clearly demonstrates that simultaneous discoveries and procedural improvements contributed to the evolution of interventional radiology. And although progress is often slow, that evolution continues.

To understand how the discoveries of the pioneers of interventional radiology came about, it is necessary to keep two factors in mind: the common knowledge (or lack thereof) that existed at the time and the financial and material resources available to the pioneers. Both were woefully limited. The laboratories of the day were not advanced by contemporary standards, and the pioneering inventors frequently had to design and build their own equipment to specifications that existed only in their imaginations.

The discoveries of the pioneers of interventional radiology forever changed the way many procedures are performed, thereby resulting in greater comfort for countless patients and the sparing of untold lives. It is to the selfless determination of these pioneers—working against painful and persistent odds—that this book is dedicated.

Tools of the Trade: Needle and Syringe Development

Imagine that you are walking barefoot along a garden path when you feel a sharp pain in your foot. You bend over to inspect your foot and discover a stinger from a squashed bee imbedded in your skin. While you are bent over removing the offending stinger, you notice the hollow tooth of a snake lying on the ground. You place both the stinger and the tooth in the palm of your hand; you are holding history. These were the first devices that ever injected foreign substances into the human body.

Granted, the insect stinger and snake tooth were not deployed with your informed consent . . . but they are quite efficient percutaneous injectors.

First Intravenous Injection

In 1665, the famed Oxford University architect and astronomer Christopher Wren performed the first recorded intravenous injection. Wren was convinced that substances could be injected directly into the veins rather than administered orally or through the rectum, which were the established procedures at that time.

Wren injected crocus metallorum (a mixture of antimony oxysulfide and antimony oxide) into some healthy large dogs and opium into other dogs of similar stature. The dogs injected with the crocus metallorum vomited to death; those injected with opium fell into a stupor. Wren had a prized opium-injected dog that grew fat and famous and was ultimately appropriated by an unknown thief, thus resulting in one of the earliest recorded cases of a scientist having his work stolen.

Johann Daniel Major popularized the idea of making intravenous injections in humans. In 1667, he described the technique in his Latin treatise "Chirurgie Infusoria" (Figure 1). His equipment consisted of a silver cannula connected to a bag that could be compressed by hand. An incision had to be made into the skin first since the cannula was rather blunt. Major's goal was to inject substances that would thin the blood because many scientists at the time believed that blood was thickened by disease. Major's primary contribution, however, was the introduction of the metal hypodermic needle. One can only speculate why he did not make use of the piston syringe, which was a well-known instrument at that time.

In addition to those who were seeking entry into the vascular system was Neuner, who in 1827 described a needle and syringe system to inject mercuric chloride into the crystalline lenses of cadaver eyes to produce cataracts for practice surgery. Unfortunately, since his report was out of the mainstream of cardiovascular thought, it went relatively unnoticed. Therefore, the search for a practical needle and syringe continued.

The Modern Hypodermic Needle and Syringe

The forerunner of the modern hypodermic needle and syringe was patented in 1841 by Zophar Jayne (Figure 2). The device was created to inject an irritant solution into a hernial sac to produce inflammation. Jayne's device was about the same size as a modern-

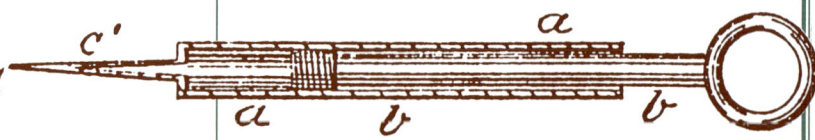

Fig. 2. The forerunner of the modern hypodermic was patented by Zophar Jayne in 1841.

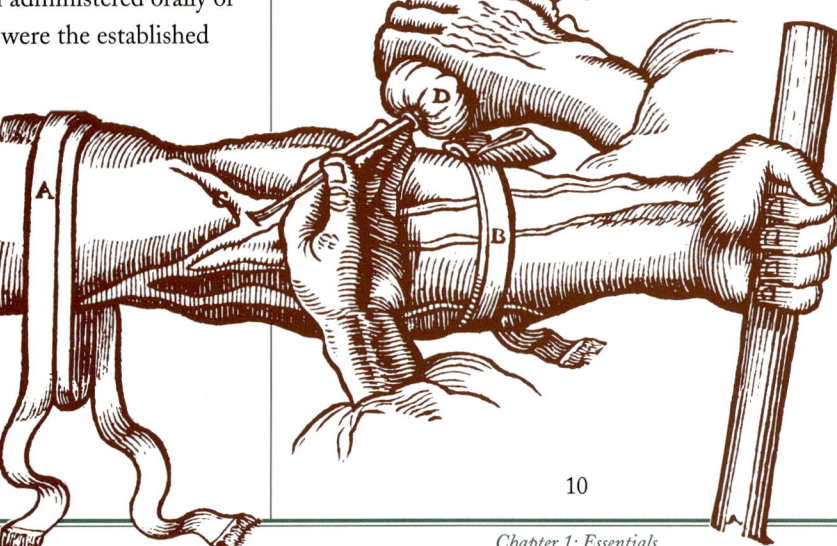

Fig. 1. Johann Daniel Major popularized intravenous injections in the mid-1600s as a method for thinning blood. His innovation was the use of a metal hypodermic needle.

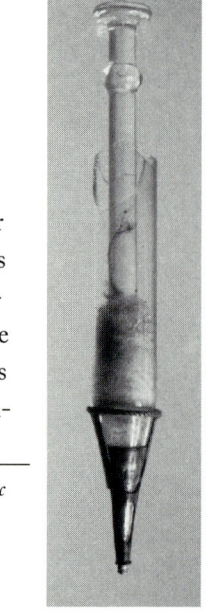

Fig. 3. The first modern steel hypodermic needle and syringe was developed by Alexander Wood around 1850.

day tuberculin syringe. The syringe was made of metal, and the permanently attached needle (or "beak") had side holes (see c' in Figure 2) that allowed the chosen fluid to escape. With the use of an airtight piston, Jayne was able to fill the barrel of his device with whatever volume of liquid he pleased.

The first to use the modern steel hypodermic needle and syringe was the Scottish physician Alexander Wood, who described his system (Figure 3) around 1850. Wood's earliest syringe, used to inject morphine subcutaneously to relieve pain in patients suffering from neuralgia, was

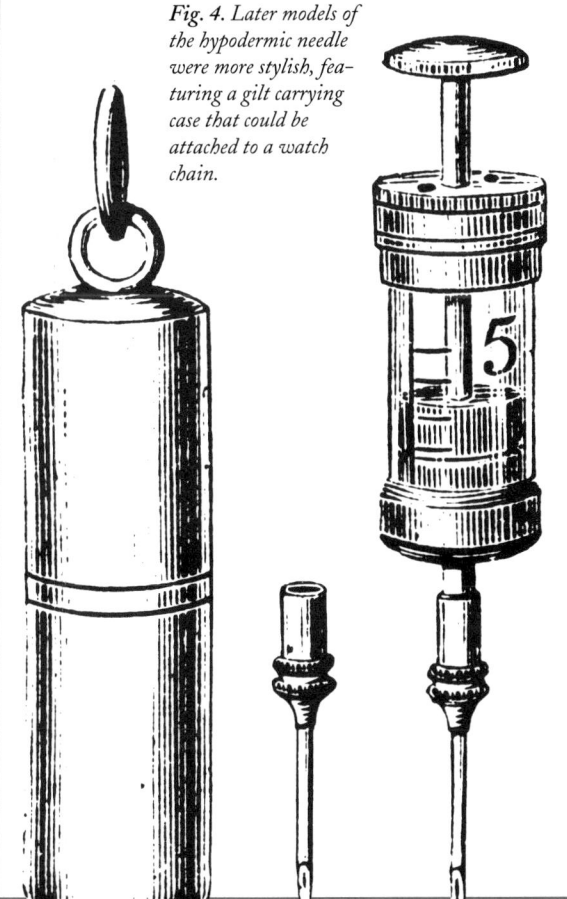

Fig. 4. Later models of the hypodermic needle were more stylish, featuring a gilt carrying case that could be attached to a watch chain.

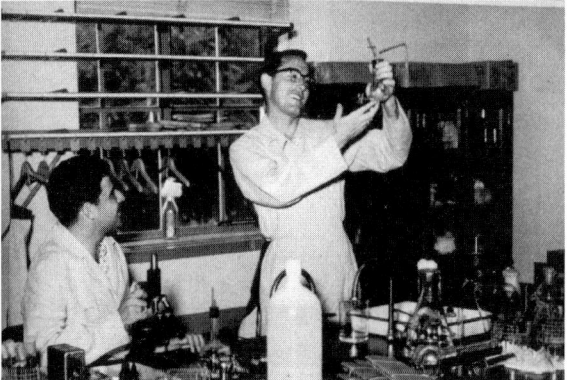

Fig. 7. Ross Jennings

made of glass and had a conical metal nose cap that held a detachable needle. The piston contained a conical tip that fit into the nose cap. His original version did not have volumetric gradations, but a later model (Figure 4) incorporated gradations and had a gilt container for the syringe and two needles. The container was attached to a loop, allowing it to be affixed to a watch chain.

Experiments designed to coagulate blood were conducted by Charles-Gabriel Pravaz at the Veterinary School in Lyon, France. In 1853, he described experiments in which a few drops of iron perchloride were injected into sheep and horses with each turn of the threaded syringe piston. Blood flow in the carotid artery was temporarily arrested in order to produce a clot. In some interventional crystal ball, Pravaz saw the possibility of applying his method to humans to induce clot formations in treating aneurysms. Perhaps because he died the same year his report was published and human subjects were not used, Pravaz did not receive due credit for his syringe and needle. French physicians started to use the "Pravaz apparatus," but soon abandoned the screw piston and adopted a glass barrel.

A leather washer served as a gasket for the barrel's piston in the early syringe. This now-impractical feature was replaced with metal pistons, which were precision ground to fit snugly into glass barrels when the need for asepsis was recognized. The Record, a metal-piston syringe and needle, was introduced by Dewitt and Herz in 1906 (Figure 5).

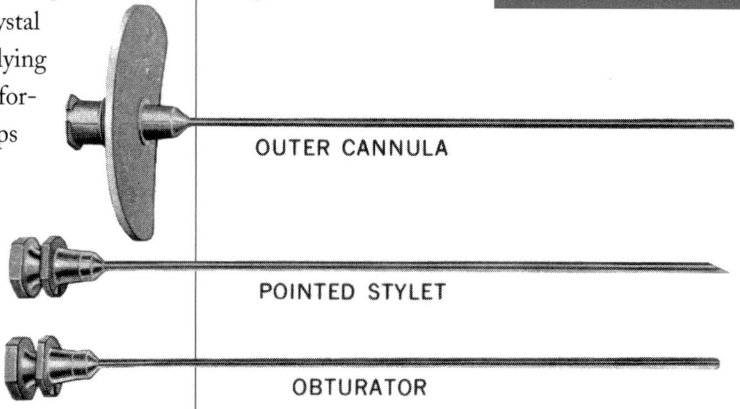

Fig. 6. Cook Incorporated's first needle, produced in 1963.

COOK'S CONTRIBUTIONS

Cook Incorporated produced its first needle in 1963. It was a stainless steel tube that enclosed a pointed stylet in the center (Figure 6).

Also in 1963, Cook introduced radiopaque Teflon tubing for catheters. Researchers from Indiana University —cardiologists Paul Lurie and Walter Judson, radiologists Eugene Klatte and Charles Helmen, and research assistant Ross Jennings (Figure 7)— developed catheterization techniques using radiopaque Teflon catheters.

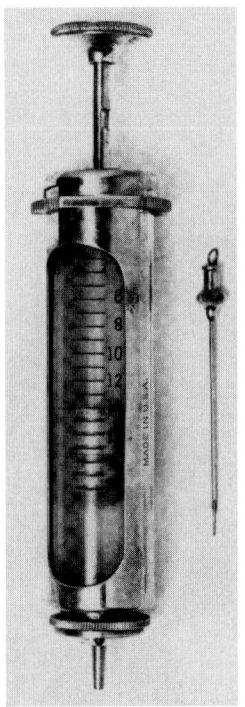

Fig. 5. In 1906, Dewitt and Herz devised the Record, a syringe with a metal piston and needle.

The All-Glass Syringe

The all-glass syringe was developed by Karl Schneider in 1896 at the Wulfing-Lüer plant in Paris (Figure 8). The Lüer catalog of 1904 reveals the concerns of the day by stating that the new syringe came with a boiling box and was "the only truly sterilizable syringe with the following advantages: (1) it is extremely simple and is easily sterilized; (2) it is not attacked by diverse alkalis, acids and oxidants; (3) has absolutely perfect graduations, assuring quantitative injections; (4) transparency of all its parts allows avoidance of the accidental injection of bubbles; and (5) the glass piston assures that the injected solution retains its purity."

The original percutaneous entry needles were produced in Sweden and consisted of an outer cannula, an inner needle, a stylet inside the inner needle, and an obturator. The obturators were the same diameter as the inner needle.

Fig. 8. Lüer introduced a syringe in 1904 that had a glass piston and barrel. Reflecting the times, advertising stressed the fact that the unit was "the only truly sterilizable syringe...."

In the United States, Becton-Dickinson produced these arterial needles in the 1940s, and subsequently the company produced a large variety of needles for direct pressure monitoring.

Becton-Dickinson also produced three-part needles, which included a needle, a stylet of identical length, and an obturator. Needle and stylet were inserted, then the stylet was pulled out. The rounded obturator tip prevented vessel gouging.

Thus, the modern sterilizable syringe and needle were available just after the beginning of the twentieth century. Percutaneous entry needles appeared shortly thereafter. However, the process of matching glass pistons and barrels, resharpening the needles, and sterilizing the equipment soon became expensive and time-consuming. These drawbacks spurred the development of the prepackaged, sterilized, disposable needles and plastic syringes that are common today.

Catheter History and Development

The word catheter is derived from the Greek word *katheter*, meaning to send down. While commonly thought to have its origins in urology, the first catheter was surely associated with the use of clysters (enemas). Used as both purgatives to restore the balance of the four humors and as a means of administering nutrients, clysters date from ancient Egyptian times, were known to Grecian medicine as early as 400 B.C., and were featured prominently in Roman

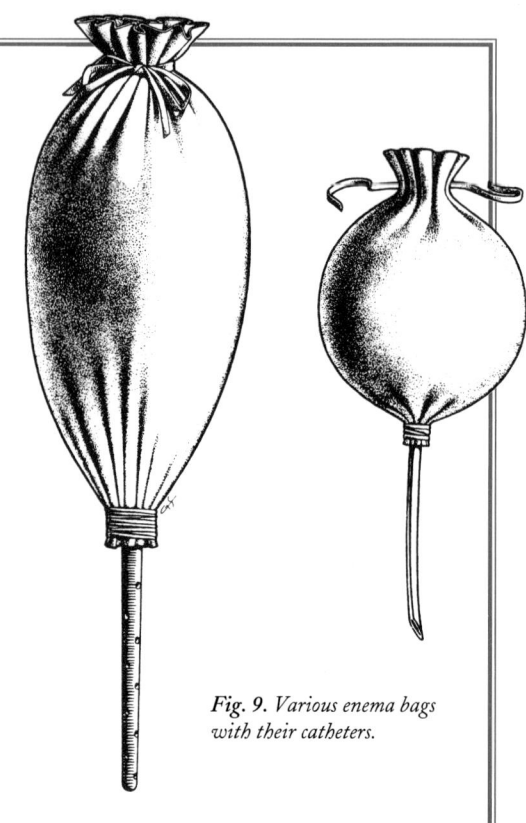

Fig. 9. Various enema bags with their catheters.

medicine at the beginning of the Christian era. The enema bag, usually an animal bladder, was affixed to a quill or metal tube, and substances were injected through the rectum by squeezing the bag (Figure 9).

Early Urologic Developments

Routine catheterization of the urinary bladder with a variety of tubes or pipes dates from Roman times. The pipes were made of lead, silver, brass, or copper, with several sizes available in both men's and women's models. Lengths were expressed in finger widths, with the macho model measuring in at 15 finger widths. Some of these tubes had a slight curve and some had a double curve. Many different catheter designs were proposed to add flexibility, yet retain enough rigidity for insertion.

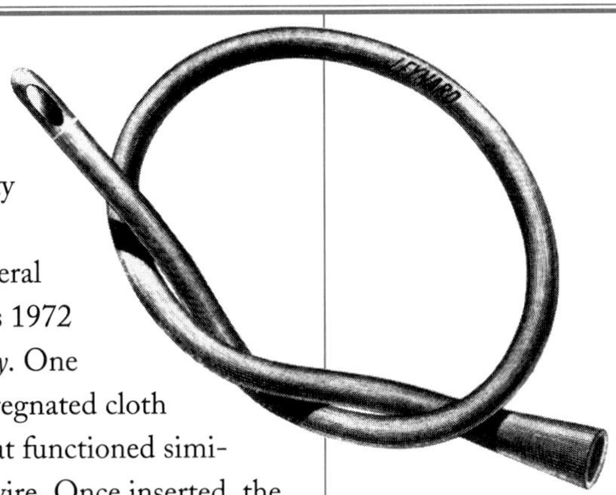

Murphy reported several early catheter designs in his 1972 book, *The History of Urology*. One design featured a wax-impregnated cloth placed over a silver tube that functioned similarly to the modern guide wire. Once inserted, the tube was withdrawn, leaving the cloth catheter in the urethra, where unfortunately, body heat softened the wax and the catheter collapsed. Another design incorporated a spiral of flat silver wire; the coils were first covered with sewn parchment and then with wax. This flexible catheter could be left in the body for several days, but was not used extensively at the time.

Urologists in the early 1800s had two primary goals: to develop a pliant, smooth, urine-resistant catheter and to devise a means of widening urethral strictures. Attempts were made by Cazenave in 1875 to fabricate catheters from highly processed whalebone or ivory (Figure 10). However, the best-known urethral catheter of the day was made by the famous surgeon Auguste Nelaton. His straight, vulcanized rubber catheter—resistant to urine—became commercially available in the late 1800s, and the urologists' first goal was met (Figure 11).

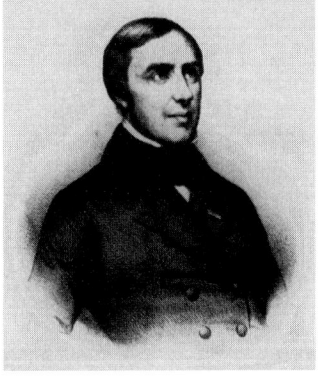
Fig. 11. Surgeon Auguste Nelaton devised a vulcanized rubber catheter, which became commercially available in the late 1800s.

Earlier in the century, in 1846, Mercier had conceived the idea of providing a single or double curve at the tip of a rubber urethral catheter, unwittingly preempting Nelaton's technology (Figure 12). Mercier created his catheter with a malleable wire stylet; numerous patient trials were necessary to establish the best curvature.

Early interventional urologists devised a variety of techniques to widen urethral strictures, which they recognized as their other primary objective. In 1846, Benique described a technique of introducing catheters with increasing diameters into the urethra (á la Dotter) and alternately using catheters with olive-shaped bulbs at their tips as dilators. Other catheters, with tapered tips and side holes, were used to inject silver nitrate to destroy stricture tissue.

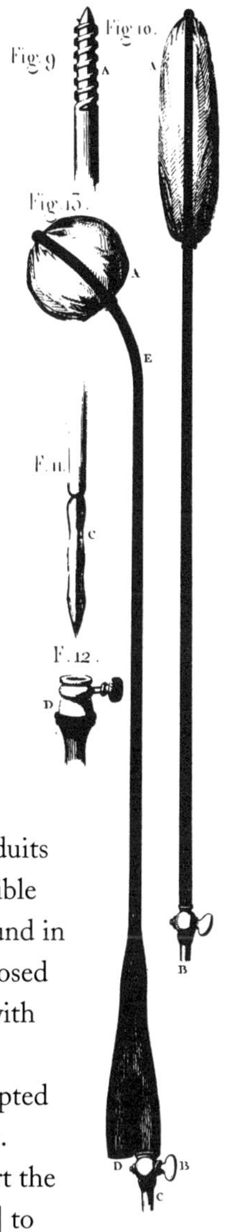

The French physician Reybard was apparently the first to develop a balloon-tipped catheter (Figure 13). In 1855, he described his preferred technique for widening strictures, which involved the use of curved and balloon-tipped catheters. Reybard provided the details of his equipment, which included a "Rubber sound [or catheter] of double lumen with two conduits on which is mounted a distensible ampoule . . . used to fix the sound in the bladder. [a] little tap . . . closed after distending the ampoule with air or water introduced with a syringe . . . [a] rubber tube adapted to the tap to facilitate injection. [and] Dilators . . . to push apart the wound after the operation, [or] to compress the engorged prostate."

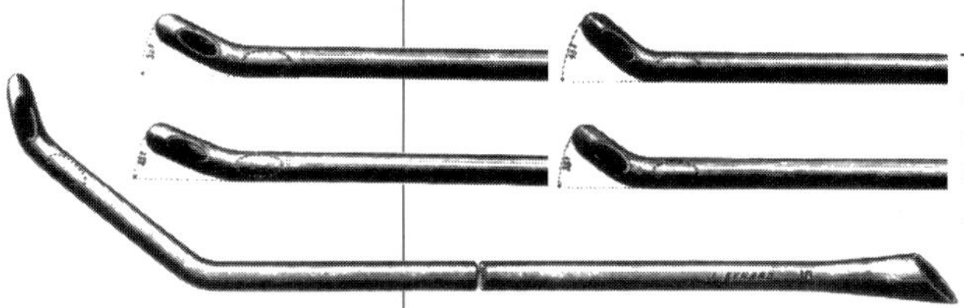

Fig. 13. Reybard is credited with developing the first inflatable, balloon-tipped urethral catheters.

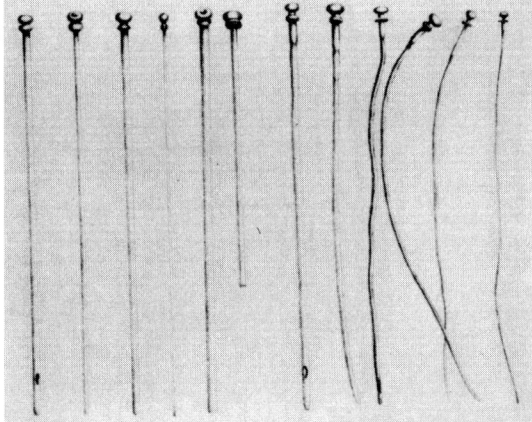
Fig. 10. Cazenave fashioned catheters from whalebone.

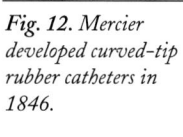
Fig. 12. Mercier developed curved-tip rubber catheters in 1846.

Chapter 1: Essentials

Although satisfactory catheters had been developed, it was difficult to retain them in the bladder for many days despite some ingenious strategies, including tying and taping the catheters in place.

Oddly, the most successful of the self-retaining, inflatable balloon-tipped catheters was developed not for retention but for hemostasis by tamponade following transurethral resection. This catheter was first described by Foley in 1929; in 1937, he discussed the catheter's drainage properties. Thus, his Foley hemostatic bag catheter, distributed by American Cystoscope Makers, Inc. (Figure 14), served a dual purpose. An inflatable water balloon was placed near the tip of the catheter; upon inflation, it arrested bleeding. In the first model, Foley affixed an inflation tube to the outside of the catheter, but a later model featured two lumens—one for balloon inflation and one for urine passage (Figure 15).

Meanwhile, others (Gerow, 1933; Belknap, 1933) described self-retaining catheters similar to Foley's. Gerow even patented his. Unfortunately, design limitations made commercial success of both catheters impossible.

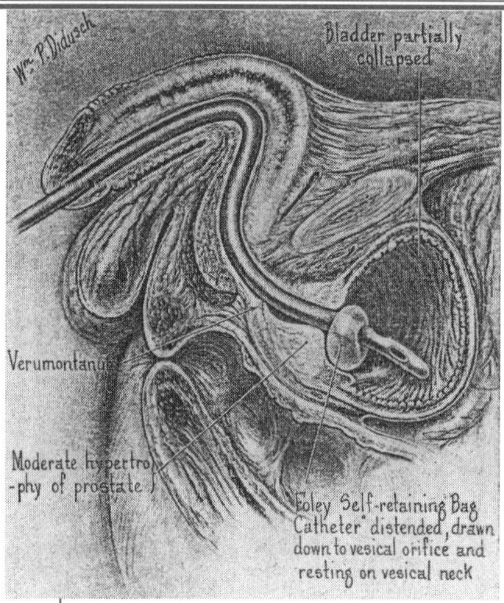

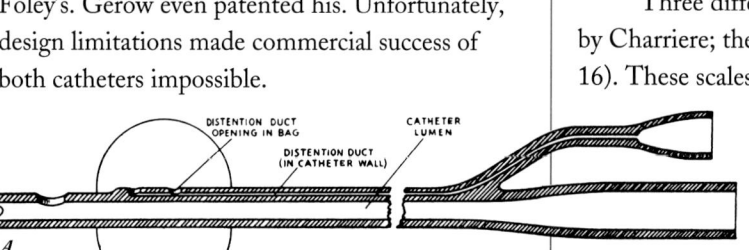

Fig. 15. This sketch of Foley's self-retaining balloon catheter shows the balloon inflated while inside the bladder. Five milliliters of sterile water were used to distend the balloon.

The French Scale

While virtually everyone in medicine is familiar with the French (F) scale, few know of its origins in urology. Widening of urethral strictures was a well-established practice by the mid-1800s. Not surprisingly, it was desirable to identify the outer diameter of catheters so that successively larger catheters could be passed into the urethra. Sir Henry Thompson provided background information about urologic catheter sizing in an 1883 publication.

Three different scales arose: the French, devised by Charriere; the English; and the Scottish (Figure 16). These scales were quite different. Charriere's was based on one-third millimeter (for example, the diameter of a Size 1 Charriere catheter is one-third millimeter). The British scale was based on fractions (1/64) of an inch. The Scottish scale, also based on inches, was coarser—one and one-half times larger than the English scale.

International controversy ensued. With sentiment atypical of the British, Sir Henry Thompson encouraged adoption of the Charriere (French) scale: "In England, we cannot be said to have a uniform scale; all our measurements are very arbitrary. . . . Our exact neighbors over the channel use the millimeter and the number itself expresses the precise size. . . . I advise you in this, and in other matters, to be cosmopolitan in your views and to adopt improvements from all quarters."

The French scale emerged victorious. When vascular catheters appeared on the scene, the French scale was conveniently applied to specify their diameters as well.

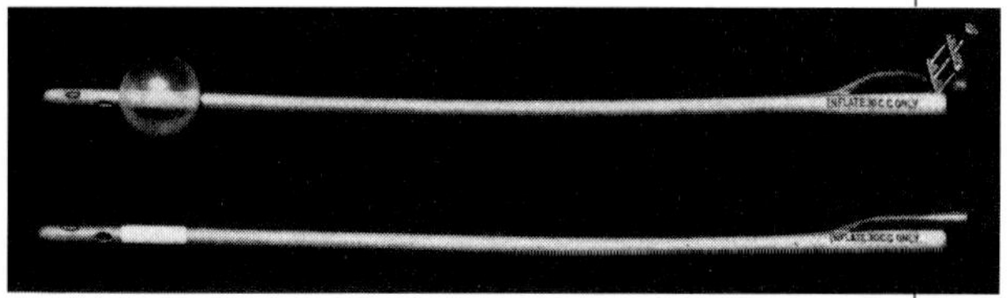

Fig. 14. These illustrations show Foley's hemostatic bag catheter. Sketch (A) shows the various components and (B) illustrates the balloon inflated and deflated.

Fig. 16. (A) This chart compares the Charriere (French) scale to the English scale. (B) is a historic French scale reproduced in miniature.

Scale of Charrière	1	2	3	4	5	6	7	8
English Scale			1			2		3
Scale of Charrière	9	10	11	12	13	14	15	16
English Scale	4	5	6		7		8	9
Scale of Charrière	17	18	19	20	21	22	23	24
English Scale	10		11		12	13		14

A

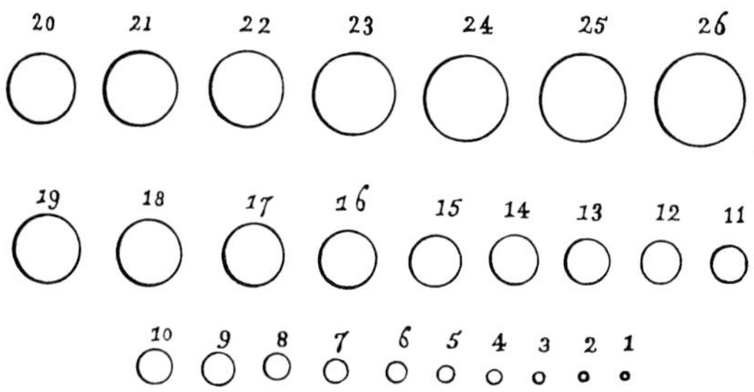

B

Vascular Catheter Developments

The first use of vascular catheters actually seems to have occurred in the mid-1600s. The earliest experiments involved the transfusion of blood from the artery of one animal into the vein of another. In London in 1667, Richard Lower conducted an experiment in which he directed carotid blood of a sheep into the jugular vein of a young man through a catheter. This first "catheter" consisted of two silver pipes—one in the sheep and one in the man—and a quill that constituted communication between the tubes.

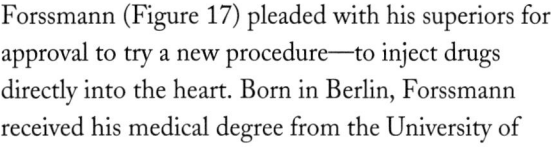

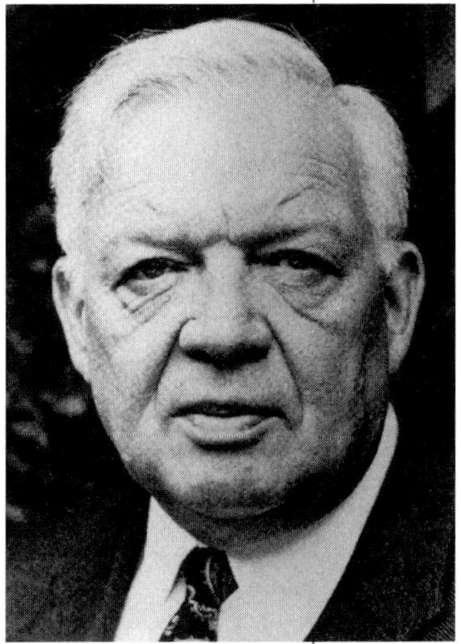

Fig. 17. Werner Forssman catheterized his own heart in 1929 to prove catheterization could be done.

Similar experiments followed, some successful and others disastrous. Blood transfusion was soon abandoned for more than two centuries until rubber tubing was finally used to collect or transfuse the blood. Still other investigations in the 1700s and 1800s used catheters to measure blood pressure. Catheter materials in these studies included glass, brass, lead, and other metals.

The use of compliant intravascular catheters dates from 1929 when Werner Forssmann (Figure 17) pleaded with his superiors for approval to try a new procedure—to inject drugs directly into the heart. Born in Berlin, Forssmann received his medical degree from the University of Berlin in 1929. That year, he interned at the Auguste Viktoria Home in Eberswalde, where stoic superiors frowned upon Forssmann's idea.

Unable to persuade others of his new concept's validity, Forssman took matters into his own hands. Using a sterile venesection kit, he made an incision in his skin. He inserted a Dechamps aneurysm needle into his right antecubital vein, opened it, and pushed a urethral catheter toward his heart. He had some x-rays taken as documentation (Figure 18). In 1931, Forssmann published a paper describing this event.

The vascular catheters advanced with Cournand's first description in 1941 of catheterization of the right atrium in a human heart in which he

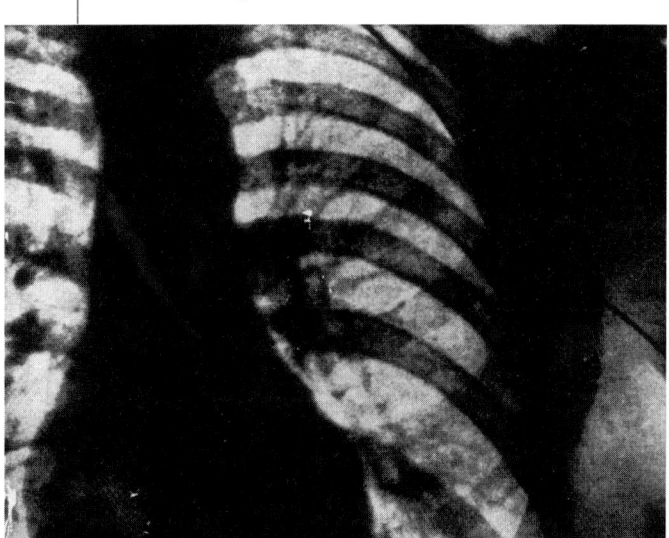

Fig. 18. X-ray of a urethral catheter in Forssman's right heart.

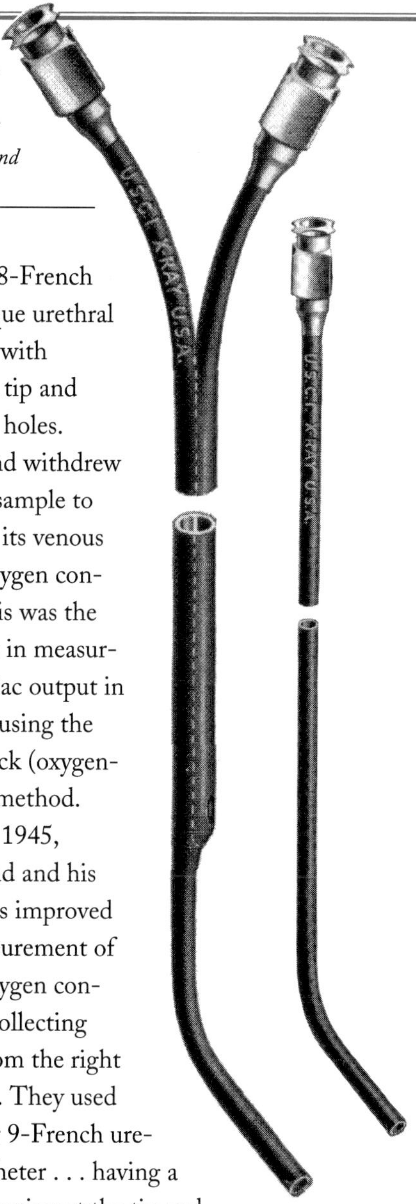

Fig. 19. Cournand devised a number of catheters and electrodes.

used an 8-French radiopaque urethral catheter with rounded tip and two side holes. Cournand withdrew a blood sample to measure its venous blood oxygen content. This was the first step in measuring cardiac output in humans using the direct Fick (oxygen-uptake) method.

In 1945, Cournand and his associates improved the measurement of blood oxygen content by collecting blood from the right ventricle. They used an "8- or 9-French urethral catheter . . . having a single opening at the tip and a special air-tight adapter at the base for a Lüer syringe." The catheter also featured a slight curve in its distal three inches to facilitate manipulation (Figure 19).

Cournand's catheter was fabricated by the United States Catheter and Instrument Corporation (USCI) of Glens Falls, New York, a company founded in 1939 by David Sheridan and Norman Jeckel. The company's cooperation—and the early availability of its vascular catheters—enabled others to measure cardiac output using the direct Fick method.

By the time Seldinger introduced his percutaneous entry technique in 1953, polyethylene tubing had made its appearance. This material could be drawn to reduce its diameter, and it would retain its shape once it had been transformed in boiling water and cooled. Unfortunately, it was not radiopaque.

The radiopaque polyethylene catheter was described in 1956 by Per Ödman, a radiologist from Karolinska Institute. Working with Ledin from Kirurgiska Instrument Fabriks Aktiebolaget (KIFA), he incorporated the salts of heavy metals into polyethylene, creating the popular Ödman-Ledin tubing that was available in three outer diameters—"red, green, and yellow" (Figure 20). KIFA provided comprehensive instructions to radiologists who heat-formed their own catheters.

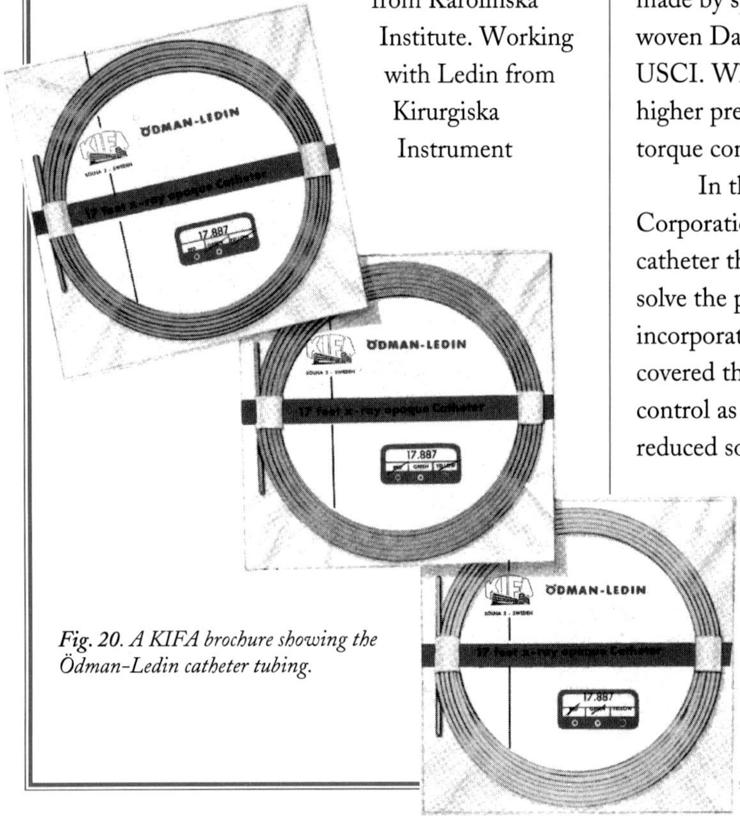

Fig. 20. A KIFA brochure showing the Ödman-Ledin catheter tubing.

High Pressure and Torque Control

Meanwhile, researchers began to recognize that considerable pressure was necessary to inject viscous contrast medium. They also realized the need to manipulate the catheter more easily into the vessel of choice. As catheters were modified to withstand high-pressure injections, the new catheters acquired another attractive feature—torque control.

Early high-pressure vascular catheters were first made by spraying varnish over nylon and later over woven Dacron. These catheters were fabricated by USCI. While the USCI catheters could withstand a higher pressure than others, they lacked adequate torque control.

In the early 1960s, Robert Stevens of Cordis Corporation (Figure 21) set out to develop the best catheter that modern technology would allow. To solve the problem of bursting under high pressure, he incorporated metal braid into catheter walls and discovered that the metal braid provided excellent torque control as well. Furthermore, the increased stiffness reduced so-called catheter whip. Stevens first fabricated his new catheter from extruded polyethylene and then from polyurethane. By milling bismuth subcarbonate into the urethane prior to extrusion, he was able to make the catheter radiopaque. No braid was present in the tip, ensuring tip softness and allowing retention of a preformed curve.

Officials from USCI saw the first prototype of Stevens' braided catheter at a meeting in Miami in March of 1963. Shortly thereafter, Stevens agreed to let USCI manufacture the catheter. But after a considerable investment of time and money, USCI was unable to produce the catheter to Stevens' satisfaction. Stevens therefore requested that the agreement be canceled, although the company continued to incorporate the braided wire into the wall of its original Positrol catheters, which had satisfactory rotational qualities but whose tips did not retain their shape well.

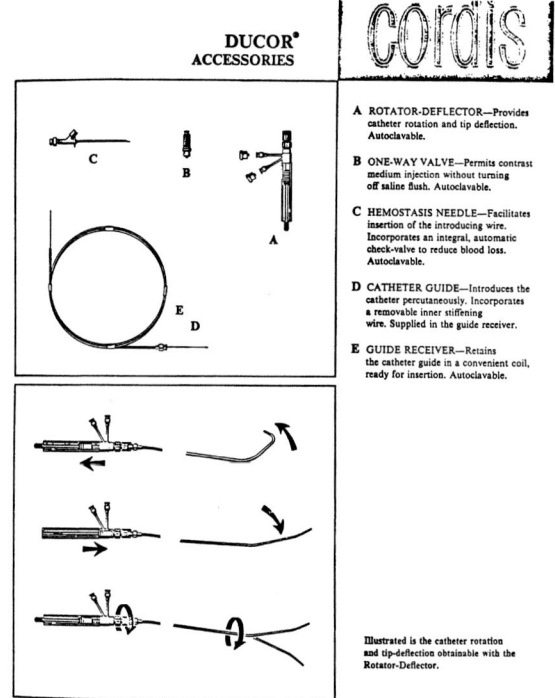

Fig. 21. The first Cordis catalog was a simple sheet of paper.

Cordis Corporation applied for patents on Stevens' catheter and received them in 1969. Cook Incorporated was the first manufacturer to copy the stainless braided catheter, and sometime later USCI copied it as well. Cook's catheter was fabricated of polyethylene; USCI's Positrol II was of polyurethane. Subsequently, many other companies acquired licenses to manufacture the Stevens metal-braided, radiopaque, preformed tip catheter.

Heparin Coating
Physicians who introduced catheters and implanted vascular grafts often encountered the problem of thrombus formation. One solution was systemic anticoagulation agents—usually heparin. This technique was not without its hemorrhagic hazards, however. In fact, the heparinization of patients was not an established procedure.

In a dramatic exchange of opinion and fact in the early 1970s, Bill Cook was accused of practicing medicine without a license at a radiology conference when he suggested the routine use of systemic heparinization in all angiographic catheterization procedures. After a vociferous uproar, Porstmann and Dotter brought a sudden end to the discussion when they told the attendees that, for quite some time, they had been using the heparin procedure Cook suggested.

Meanwhile, efforts were under way in the late 1960s and early 1970s to develop a process by which heparin could be bonded to vascular catheters and implant surfaces. These chemical processes varied in complexity and effectiveness. In 1971, Amplatz developed a simple method of rendering plastic surfaces antithrombogenic with a benzalkonium heparin coating that did not strip off during percutaneous insertion and delayed thrombus formation up to four hours in canine tests. The Amplatz method is used on some Cook Incorporated catheters and wire guides; several other manufacturers supply antithrombogenic devices, as well.

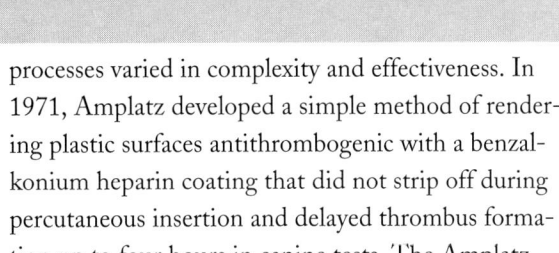

Fig. 22. Cook Incorporated produced catheter sheaths made of Mylar in the mid-1960s.

Sheaths as Introducers
Angiographic catheterization procedures became more common and more demanding throughout the 1960s and 1970s. The use of closed-tipped and balloon-tipped catheters necessitated an "introducer" to facilitate entry into the vascular system. To gain access to the vessel using percutaneous entry techniques, physicians began to introduce a dummy catheter (or dilator) over which was placed a thin-walled sheath. When the dummy catheter was removed, the specialized catheter (closed- or balloon-tipped, for example) could be introduced easily through the sheath.

The Desilets-Hoffman catheter introducers were a major contribution to the placement of specialized catheters into the vascular system. Created by Donald Desilets and Richard Hoffman from UCLA (with help from Herbert Ruttenberg), the first sets of catheter sheaths were homemade from DuPont Mylar soda straws. In 1965, Cook Incorporated began commercial production of the Desilets-Hoffman introducer (Figure 22). The early sets were fabricated from Mylar straws, too. Later, in 1969, a thin-walled Teflon sheath replaced the straw.

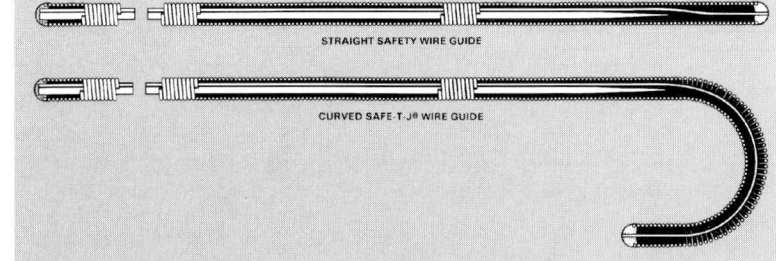

Fig. 23. A major advance in wire guides came with Cook's introduction of the safety wire.

A GIANT LEAP FORWARD

Wire-guide evolution took a dramatic leap forward when Cook Incorporated introduced the safety wire in 1965. Melvin Judkins' work with these wires in 1967 popularized the safety feature. The guides had an internal wire running from tip to tip. The wire kept coils from elongating or, worse, breaking off within the vessel. Judkins used Cook's Teflon-coated Safe-T-J wires (Figure 23) and specially shaped Cordis Ducor polyurethane catheters in his novel technique—selective coronary artery catheterization.

Wire Guide Evolution

In their quest to direct a catheter into the vascular system and guide its course, researchers turned to a remarkable variety of wires, cables, and other equipment. They faced a dilemma, however: how to insert a catheter significantly larger in diameter than their needle into the vessel. Surgical cutdown of the vessel was an established procedure; furthermore, the Mayo Clinic and other medical centers used a procedure in which a catheter was inserted through a needle. Seldinger, seeking another mode of entry, initially used an ordinary silver wire ("leader") in his experiments, eventually settling upon a hand-coiled wire guide. He, like many early angiographers, made his own guides by purchasing wire from machine shops and coiling it by hand or on lathes. Others, such as Dotter, used more creative materials—piano and guitar strings and speedometer cables, for example.

KIFA of Sweden manufactured the first "wire guides according to Seldinger" and offered them for sale along with catheter tubing and hand-fabrication tools. Schick X-Ray of Chicago distributed these KIFA materials in the United States (Figure 24). The first commercially available guide wires had a fixed core.

Charles Dotter brought a moveable-core wire guide to the United States from Europe, where the idea originated. In 1963, Cook Incorporated became the first domestic manufacturer of this improved guide. The handle enabled the center core to be moved and allowed flexibility by varying the length of the tip (Figure 25).

At Cook Incorporated, the use of lathes to coil guide wires gave way to the use of a highly modified Torrington coiler in the early 1960s. In 1966, Cook's Tom Osborne (Figure 26) invented a secret process for coiling, referred to as the Osborne process, that the company still uses. Osborne was in his late teens at the time. Some manufacturers still use the lathe-coiling technique.

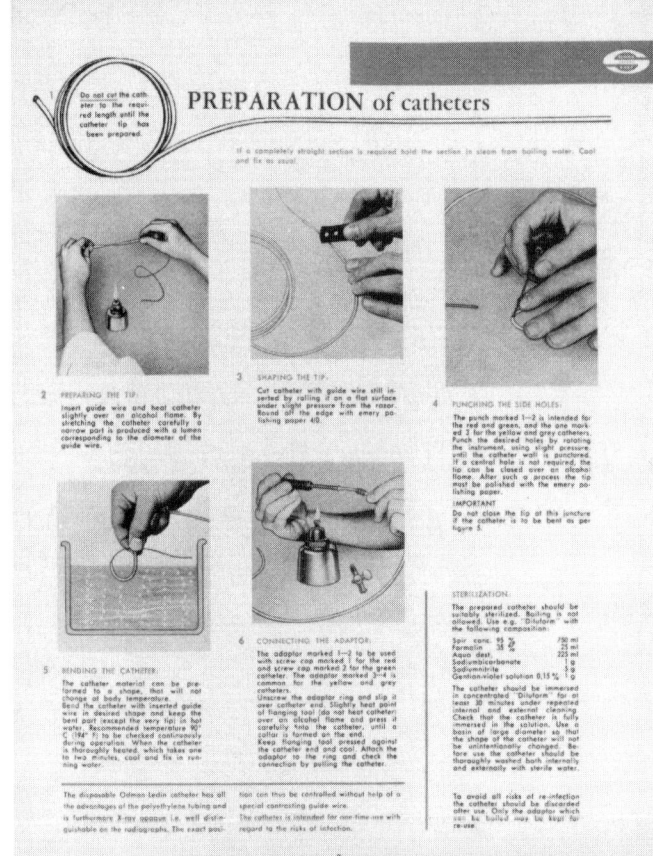

Fig. 24. Schick X-Ray of Chicago distributed KIFA products. The catalog included instructions on how to form catheters.

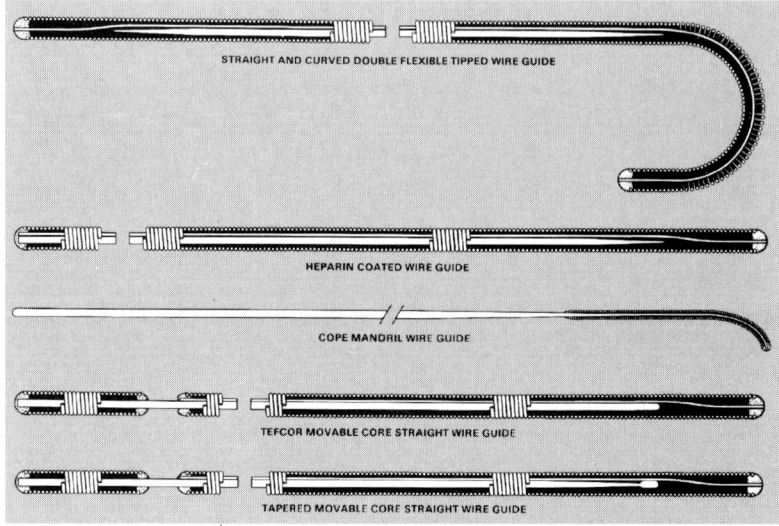

Fig. 25. Over the last thirty years, Cook Incorporated has developed a variety of wire guides.

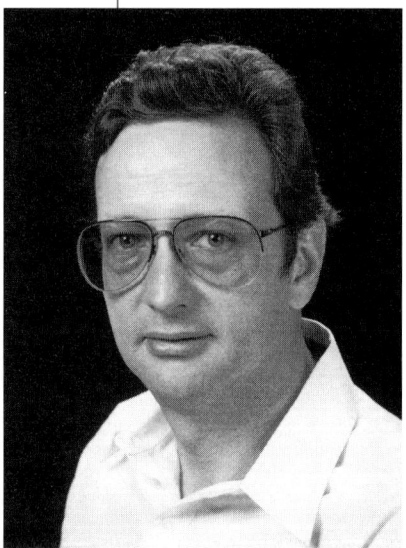

Fig. 26. Tom Osborne

Catheter-tip straighteners and tip deflectors soon evolved from the guide wire. The first commercially produced controllable tip deflector (developed in the early 1960s) was USCI's Muller Tip Deflecting System, which allowed the user to steer the catheter in a number of different directions (Figure 27). Cordis Corporation introduced the Roto-Flector tip-straightening system shortly thereafter. In 1966, Cook Incorporated developed a tip-deflecting system for Stuart Reuter. Medi-Tech then introduced its deflector, not for use in blood vessels but in the bronchial tree and gastrointestinal tract (Figure 28).

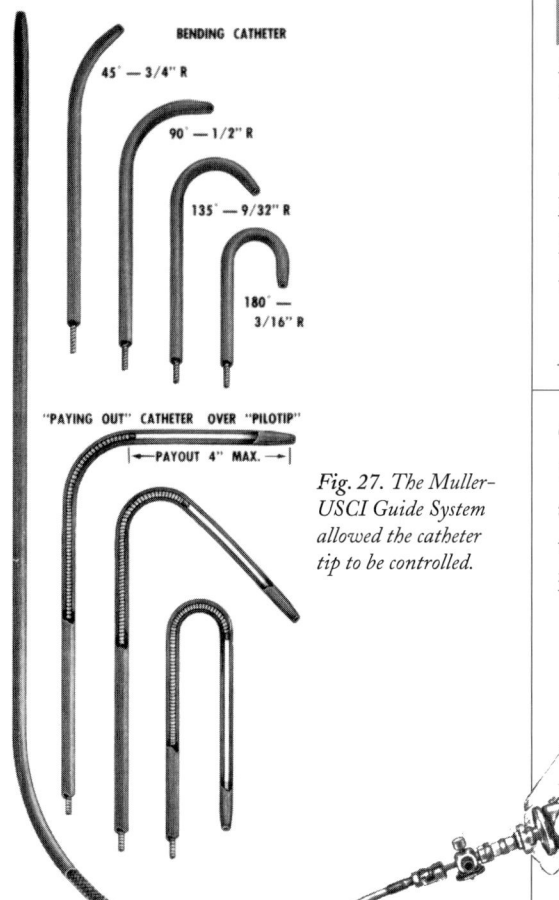

Fig. 27. The Muller-USCI Guide System allowed the catheter tip to be controlled.

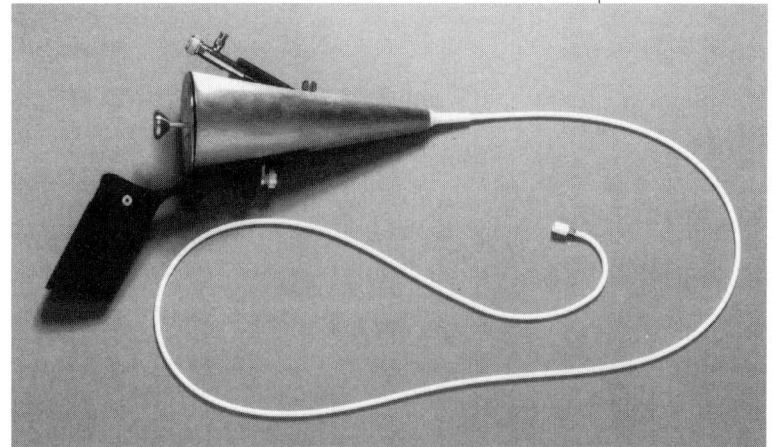

Fig. 28. Medi-Tech introduced a steerable catheter for use in the bronchial tree and gastrointestinal tract.

X-ray Imaging Improvements

On November 8, 1895, Wilhelm Conrad Roentgen (Figure 29), professor of physics at Würzburg, applied high voltage to the electrodes of a Crookes tube. In his darkened lab, he noticed a glow emanating from some nearby barium platinocyanide crystals. He designated his rays "x" and set about examining their properties. Neither a thick book nor tinfoil would block Roentgen's rays, but sheets of gold, platinum, and lead provided varying degrees of absorption. The rays also darkened unexposed photographic plates, and a human hand applied to a plate covered with fluorescent salts cast an eerie shadow of the bones (Figure 30).

Image Intensifiers

Roentgen's experiments were soon duplicated throughout the world, and by the early 1930s, the diagnostic x-ray machine had reached a high degree of sophistication. In 1912, Eastman Kodak introduced the first plates specially created for radiology. Efforts aimed at producing high-quality motion pictures of x-ray images began as early as 1921 and continued through the age of video.

Others sought ways to brighten x-ray images with image intensifiers, allowing practical cinefluorography without requiring high current and high voltage. The first device was patented by Coolidge in 1939; it was used with a conventional fluoroscopic screen. Langmuir then patented the forerunner of the modern image intensifier in 1940, incorporating a fluorescent screen into the device.

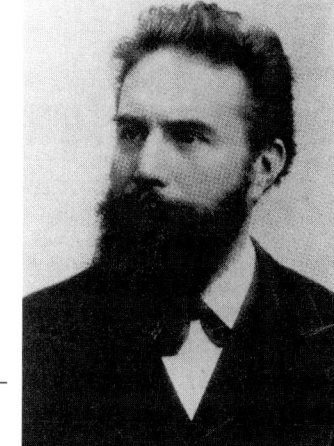

Fig. 29. Wilhelm Roentgen discovered x-rays in 1895.

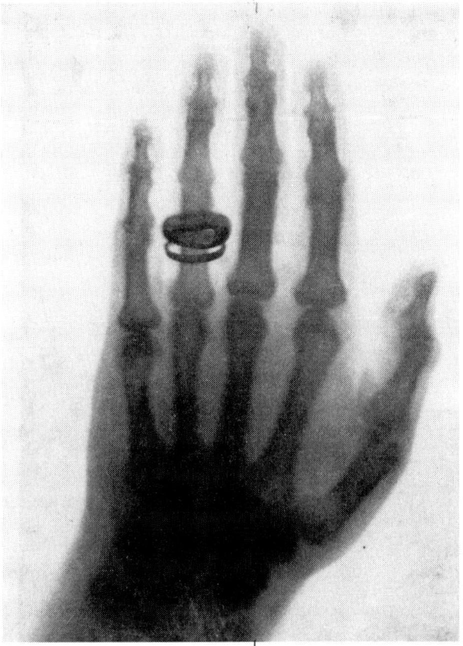

Fig. 30. Roentgen took this x-ray of the hand of Kolliker, professor of anatomy at Würzburg.

Image intensifiers were commercially available in the early 1950s, but they did not permit simultaneous viewing and photography. Investigators themselves added these features, as well as television monitoring. Manufacturers quickly followed suit.

Contrast Media

Published reports from Haschek and Lindenthal in 1896 and Cannon in 1898 demonstrated early that imaging of the vascular system and hollow organs was possible using x-ray-absorbing contrast medium. Investigations conducted from 1918 to 1923 led to the conclusion that iodides of potassium and sodium absorb x-rays and could be appropriate contrast media. The stage was set for vascular imaging.

Among the first to use sodium iodide for angiography were Berberich and Hirsch in 1923 and Brooks in 1924. Brooks injected sodium iodide into the femoral artery and visualized the popliteal and posterior tibial arteries (Figure 31). Because the primary therapy for vascular occlusion in a limb was amputation at that time, the development of vascular imaging began to assume greater importance.

The search for an adequate contrast medium continued through the 1920s, 1930s, and 1940s. Sicard and Forestier reported the first use of iodinated poppy seed oil (Lipiodol) in 1923. Four years later, Moniz discovered that, though possessing excellent opacity, thorium dioxide became radioactive when bombarded with x-rays. During the 1930s, both sodium iodide and iodinated organic compounds were the primary media of choice. Several investigators (Nuvoli, 1936; Reyboul and Racine, 1936; and others) injected media directly into the left ventricle and ascending aorta in humans. Hazards of arrhythmia, hemorrhage, and pneumothorax discouraged many from using this technique.

Jönsson pointed out in a 1948 study that in order to obtain good arteriograms, the tip of the catheter delivering contrast media should be at the aortic valve. Although Jönsson designated his paper a preliminary report, it marked the beginning of modern coronary angiography. Many other researchers soon reported their techniques, ranging from the use of acetylcholine to temporarily arrest the heart to the use of a looped catheter within the aorta.

Regardless of the differences in techniques, high viscosity and high osmolality caused two undesirable results from contrast media until the mid-1970s. High-viscosity agents required the use of high pressure to inject the agents rapidly. High osmolality—the result of a high iodine content—caused several adverse responses, including an unpleasant peripheral sensation in the patient.

Almen pointed out in 1969 that non-iodine compounds could be produced to yield a low-osmolality soluble contrast agent. He was correct. Today there can be no doubt of the value of the newer contrast agents. All one needs to do is ask a patient who has experienced both media. Charles Dotter did just that in his famous "Pain and Peripheral Arteriography" studies in 1982. The widely differing patient reactions generated by the two agents are truly a study in contrasts.

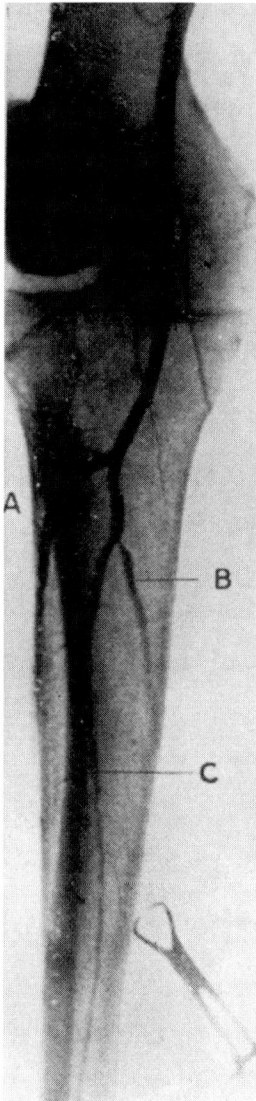

Fig. 31. Brooks obtained one of the earliest sodium iodide angiograms in 1924. He injected sodium iodide into a femoral artery to visualize the popliteal (A), popliteal (B), and posterior tibial (C) arteries.

Summary

This overview condenses centuries of medical breakthroughs, stopping for a longer look at the most important developments that affected interventional radiologists then and now. These breakthroughs did not occur automatically. They were the result of the tireless efforts of individuals striving to invent essential equipment, to perfect existing procedures, and at all times to improve the quality of life for millions of people they would never meet.

The following chapters look at some of the important pioneers in the field of interventional radiology—to see them as individuals, to uncover the sources of their inspiration, to view their motivation to solve the problems they faced, and to look at the battles they fought to gain acceptance for their new ideas. And now, meet the Catheter Introducers.

Genius is the ability to see things invisible, to manipulate things intangible, to paint things that have no features.

Joseph Joubert

CHAPTER 2: Sven Ivar Seldinger

Charting a New Course

To the angiographer, Seldinger's 1953 discovery of the percutaneous technique for inserting catheters into blood vessels is a historic breakthrough of mammoth proportions. By sailing over the edge of established medical practice with nothing but a thin-walled introducer needle, a wire guide, and a preformed catheter as his ship to adventure, Sven Seldinger discovered a whole new world of possibilities for angiographers—a world that quickened the medical profession and inspired many other members of the radiology community to embark on exploratory missions of their own.

Seldinger (Figure 1) did not publish much, but that did not seem to matter. He proved that the quality of publication is more important than quantity by announcing his discovery through a brief and concise nine-page article (including pictures) in the May 1953 edition of the Scandinavian medical journal *Acta Radiologica*. In his report, "Catheter Replacement of the Needle in Percutaneous Arteriography," Seldinger writes, "This technique is simpler than it appears on paper and after a little practice should present no difficulties."

Learned by Observing
The Seldinger technique was so uncomplicated that many early radiologists simply learned how to perform the procedure by watching someone else do it. In fact, Charles Dotter and Melvin Judkins were among those who learned the technique through reading and observation.

Dotter addressed the simplicity of the method and its impact by stating, "Seldinger will not be forgotten. His technique is a medical milestone, which illuminates the major significance that can attend an apparently simple step forward."

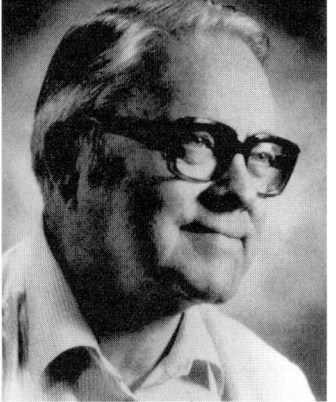

Fig. 1. Sven Ivar Seldinger in 1984.

Seldinger did not set out to discover the percutaneous entry technique. It came about as one of those miraculous sudden insights that is neither expected nor anticipated. Seldinger described the fortuitous event that changed the course of angiography in this way:

"I had the polyethylene catheter, the cannula, and the wire guide. I had made several attempts to place the catheter into a frozen cadaver aorta. And suddenly, in a split second, there came an attack of common sense. The sequence in which these three items ought to be used suddenly became obvious." Seldinger thus became the first to take the three instruments and put them together.

The Voyage to Percutaneous Catheterization

In his 1953 article, Seldinger described the work of earlier practitioners who contributed to his knowledge and paved the way for his famous discovery. He faced the same problem that presented itself to all doctors who tried to introduce a catheter into a patient's vascular system: how to do it without performing a cut-down procedure. At that time, the cut-down was the most widely used method of placing a catheter in an artery before guiding it to the desired location and injecting contrast medium.

Seldinger cited a 1941 report in which Fariñas visualized the abdominal aorta by first surgically exposing the femoral artery under local anesthesia, then puncturing the artery with a trocar and passing a catheter through it into the aorta, where contrast medium was deposited.

He also gave credit to Radner's 1947 paper describing surgical exposure of the radial artery in the forearm and passage of a catheter into it. (The distal radial artery was ligated to prevent blood loss.) Radner advanced the catheter to permit visualization of the vertebral arteries with the injected contrast medium. The distal radial artery remained ligated and collateral circulation provided blood supply to the distal regions. After he performed the vertebral angiography, Radner went on to perform thoracic aortography.

Seldinger was also inspired by Jönsson's 1941 report describing the use of a double cannula to percutaneously puncture the right common carotid artery for thoracic aortography. The outer cannula had a blunt tip while the inner cannula was shaped like a hypodermic needle. When blood issued from the inner cannula, Jönsson removed the inner cannula and passed a silver wire through the outer cannula and into the aorta, after which he advanced the cannula over the wire and into the aorta, where he injected contrast medium to visualize the aorta. The procedure was abandoned when it was feared the metal cannula might injure the aortic wall.

Puncturing Arteries Around the World

Prior to Seldinger's discovery of the percutaneous catheterization technique, several investigators wrote about their success in using a needle to puncture an artery and advance the catheter through the needle and into the vessel. In 1951, using local anesthesia, Donald and associates punctured the common carotid artery with a large bore needle that contained a stylet. After they removed the stylet, Donald and his colleagues passed the catheter into the needle and advanced it toward the head. At the desired site, the researchers injected Thorotrast to permit visualization of the cerebral vessels. Because the needle had a large bore, the process was limited to large arteries; a 1951 attempt by Peirce to catheterize the brachial artery was not promising. The process damaged the artery and held the possibility that the artery could hemorrhage after the needle was removed, since the hole in the artery was bigger than the diameter of the catheter.

Also in 1951, Bierman and associates placed 6- to 9-French catheters with permanent curves at the tips into surgically exposed carotid and radial arteries. After advancing radiopaque catheters under fluoroscopic guidance, they were able to visualize the celiac, intercostal, lumbar, and hepatic arteries by the injection of contrast medium. They used heparin to retard clotting. Interestingly, they tested the suitability of the carotid artery as a selective catheterization site before the procedure by noting its response to noninvasive occlusion. Bierman wrote, "Periodic compression of the carotid for ten minutes, three times each day, should be attained without symptoms as a prophylactic against hemiplegia [paralysis of one side of the body]."

In 1952, Rappaport devised a catheter guide consisting of a tightly coiled wire wound around a straight wire and joined at the tip. The straight wire could be placed under tension by turning a nut on the end, causing the coiled wire to "bend like a candy cane." The straight guide was then placed in a catheter that was advanced by cut-down of the femoral artery. Under fluoroscopic examination, Rappaport advanced both the catheter and guide to the desired aortic site. He applied tension to the guide to curve the catheter tip, which he then placed in the desired aortic branch. Once the tip was in place, he released tension, withdrew the guide, and injected contrast medium.

In 1951, Tillander described a different approach to guiding a catheter tip to a desired vascular site. He devised a catheter with gold-plated, magnetized, ball-and-socket segments at its tip. Each segment permitted 20 degrees of angular deflection. A strong external magnetic field, produced by a 200-kg electromagnet, allowed Tillander to guide the catheter tip under fluoroscopic examination. He tested the device on dogs and cadavers and found that the catheter tip could be placed in the branches of the abdominal aorta using the left radial artery as the introduction site.

The Pieces Fall Together
It was clear that someone needed to put the pieces of the puzzle together. The ingredients for the Seldinger technique existed before 1953. Fariñas, Donald, and Peirce had passed catheters through needles, and Jönsson had guided a percutaneously-inserted needle into the aorta using a silver wire.

Seldinger realized that since it was necessary to inject about 30 ml of contrast in a few seconds, a large bore catheter was needed. However, he also realized that the "catheter through the needle" and "catheter over the needle" techniques were unsuitable for large bore catheters.

In attempting to solve the problem of injecting large quantities of contrast medium into a vessel rapidly, Seldinger first tried a catheter with a side hole located a short distance from the tip. He placed a needle into the hole, with the needle tip protruding from the catheter tip (Figure 2). The needle punctured the skin and the vessel wall. Once the catheter was in place, Seldinger pushed the catheter forward into the vessel and then withdrew the needle.

Seldinger felt that, even though the method worked well, it required a skilled operator and was not suitable for catheterization of smaller vessels. He perceived other drawbacks as well. Nevertheless, he successfully used the side-hole technique for angiography to diagnose a hypernephroma, although he tried to improve the technique after a particularly difficult case.

Seldinger knew that the catheter tip had to be shaped so that it could easily enter the vessel. At first he placed a tapered metal tip on the catheter; however, because he was afraid the tip could come off in the vessel, he soon began tapering the catheter itself.

He also recognized the importance of using a wire guide, which he referred to as a leader. He fashioned his own coiled wire guides by spiral-winding a steel wire around a straight steel wire.

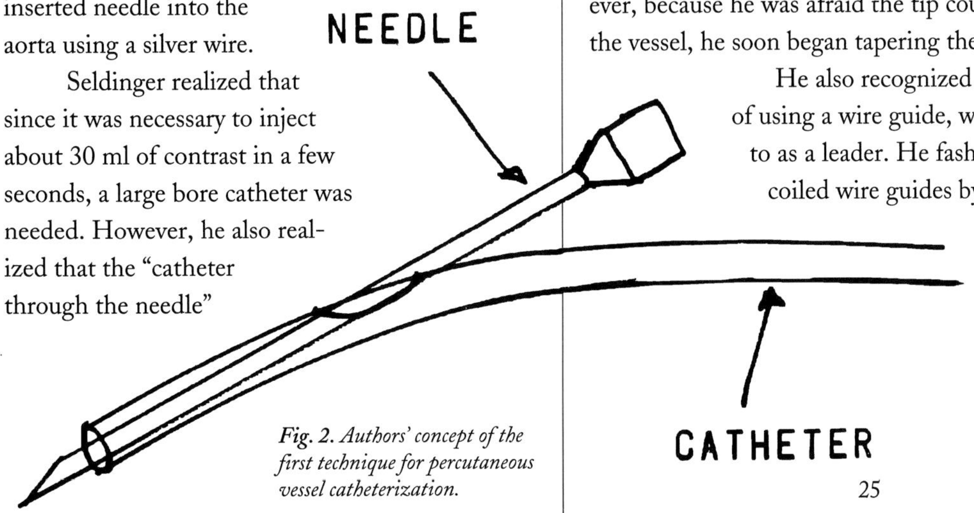

Fig. 2. Authors' concept of the first technique for percutaneous vessel catheterization.

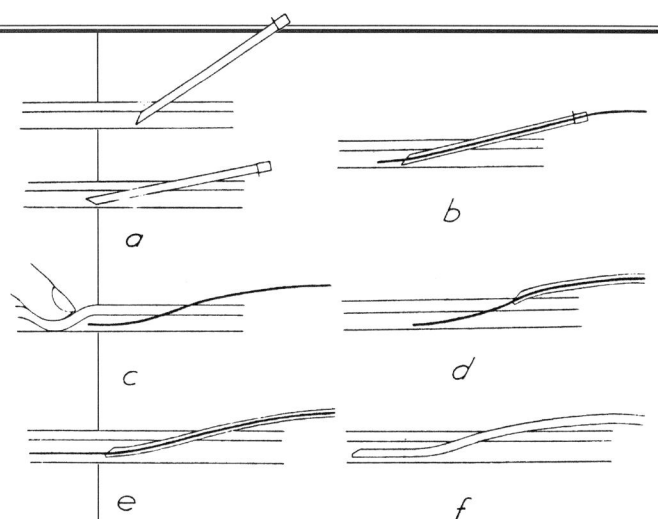

Fig. 3. This illustration appeared in Seldinger's original paper on percutaneous catheterization.

Seldinger Describes His Technique
In discussing his sudden realization of how to put all the components together, Seldinger compared his inspiration to being "similar to that of an angler—it's a bite, and it's a big fish. Hold on until he is ashore. This fight lasted the remaining 59 seconds of a minute." He also told the authors, "I can perform the procedure faster than you can write about it. Needle in, wire in, needle out, catheter over wire, wire out; that is all." Figure 3 illustrates these simple steps, for which Seldinger wrote the following instructions:

a) After local anesthesia, the artery is punctured percutaneously at a relatively small angle. After puncture, it is best to rotate the needle 180 degrees and push it a little into the artery using the bleeding as a guide to ensure that the needle remains in the artery. Puncture of arteries smaller than the femoral artery is facilitated by using an

SPEAKING ABOUT CUT-DOWNS

Prior to Seldinger's 1953 report, many cardiologists (and other physicians) inserted catheters for heart studies. Even after the introduction of the percutaneous entry technique, the cut-down mode of entry was still in use, as in the Sones technique for coronary angiography. However, it was not widespread practice for a radiologist trained in the Seldinger technique to require the service of a surgeon to perform a cut-down procedure to expose a vessel.

This circumstance may have led Sidney Wallace to remark, "The definition of interventional radiology is where the radiologist intervenes between the surgeon and his pocketbook."

---

inner needle as a guide over which the outer needle is directed into the artery.

b) The supple tip of the leader is inserted a very short distance into the lumen of the artery through the needle.

c) The leader is held in place and the needle is removed. At this moment, bleeding should be controlled by pressure on the artery proximal to the puncture site because the diameter of the leader is smaller than the hole in the artery.

d) The catheter is threaded onto the leader. When the tip reaches the skin, the free end of the leader must protrude from the catheter.

e) The catheter and leader are gripped near the skin through which they are inserted. The catheter enters the artery easily as an opening has already been made by the needle. The catheter and leader are pushed just far enough to ensure that the tip of the former is in the lumen of the vessel.

f) The leader is removed and the catheter directed to the level required, after good arterial bleeding through the catheter has been obtained. The unsupported catheter is usually pushed up the vessel without difficulty, but occasionally the leader must be re-introduced into the catheter in order to support it. The leader should not be passed beyond the tip of the catheter.

Seldinger Technique Introduced

Seldinger used his newly devised percutaneous entry technique to inject contrast medium to diagnose a parathyroid adenoma. (He claimed to the authors that his initial success was beginner's luck.) Knut Lindholm, editor of *Acta Radiologica*, wanted to mention Seldinger's new technique during the discussion of a paper at the 1952 Congress of the Northern Association of Medical Radiology, held in Helsinki. The paper to be discussed was withdrawn, but Lindholm did mention Seldinger's method and results during the discussion of another paper.

Seldinger submitted his formal paper to *Acta Radiologica* on October 28, 1952, and it was subsequently published in Volume 39 in May of 1953.

The percutaneous entry technique was used routinely at the Karolinska Hospital in Sweden, where Seldinger studied and worked for a time, but it was not initially used at the nearby Serafina, where the "catheter through needle" method was still in use. At a 1953 international surgical meeting, Seldinger presented a lecture on the percutaneous puncture of kidney cysts, covering the radiologic differentiation between renal cancer and cysts and pointing out that a cyst could be aspirated with his technique.

Many surgeons, perhaps feeling a little territorial, were less than enthusiastic about using the percutaneous entry approach instead of surgical cut-down but after about two years the technique was widely practiced in Europe. It took longer to reach the United States.

The U-Shaped Catheter

In a 1985 interview at his home in Mora, Sweden, Seldinger spoke about his percutaneous entry technique. He said his greatest surprise, relative to the method, was its widespread use for selective angiography. He did not foresee routine catheterization of very small distal vessel branches, nor did he anticipate other types of interventional radiology. This development (visualization of small vessels) became possible after the introduction of the image amplifier, a device that did not exist when Seldinger started his work.

Sodium iodide was the first contrast medium Seldinger used. The tri-iodized compounds caused very little trouble, but low osmolar compounds of the metrizamide type, such as Amipaque or Omnipaque, were a definite improvement.

While exploring applications for the percutaneous entry technique, Seldinger developed a curved catheter for selective angiography of arteries leading from the aorta. The catheter was U-shaped at one end—a radical idea for the day. This was a major discovery, but he has rarely received credit for it, probably because it was overshadowed by his discovery of the Seldinger technique.

Selective Catheterization with the U-Shaped Catheter

By the 1950s, angiographers wished to visualize small vessels, but to do so required placing a catheter tip at the vessel site and injecting contrast medium.

The techniques devised by Bierman, Tillander, and Rappaport in the early years of the decade paved the way for Seldinger's development of a U-shaped catheter, described in a 1956 paper written with Edholm and titled "Percutaneous Catheterization of the Renal Arteries." Edholm and Seldinger pointed out that it had been difficult for angiographers to control the distribution of the contrast medium. They wrote, "By injection directly into the renal artery, an amount of contrast medium adequate for examination of the kidney in question may be chosen. The difficulty in controlling the distribution of the medium by aortic injection is eliminated and the contralateral kidney preserved from any supply of contrast medium is especially valuable in the numerous cases where the kidney examined is to be removed."

Seldinger and Edholm went on to cite previous literature on the use of guided catheters and stated that the selective catheterization of a renal artery could be performed percutaneously using the following three items: "(1) a puncture needle, (2) a flexible metal guide and (3) a polyethylene catheter of the same gauge as the needle or somewhat larger."

The catheter was bent (Figure 4A) and the perpendicular distance from the tip to the straight part was somewhat larger than the diameter of the aorta. The bending was done by cautiously warming the catheter over a lighted match. The distal 3 cm of the guide was more flexible than the rest. Consequently, when the guide was introduced into the lumen of the catheter and extended 3 cm beyond its tip, the curvature of the catheter straightened (Figure 4B). When the guide was withdrawn, the catheter bent back into position. If desired, the flexible tip of the guide could remain in the curvature of the catheter to serve as a radiopaque indicator.

"After puncture, the needle is replaced by the catheter with the help of the guide," Seldinger and Edholm continued. "The guide and catheter, with the curvature straightened out, are pushed up into the aorta to the level of the renal artery. The extremity of the guide is withdrawn to the tip of the catheter, causing the latter to become curved [Figure 5]. Under fluoroscopy, the catheter is placed with its tip towards the desired kidney and is moved along the aortic wall. When it reaches the renal artery, the tip of the catheter moves outside the lateral border of the aorta. This movement was strikingly apparent in most of our cases." They reported that the catheter passed easily into the aorta during positioning.

Seldinger and Edholm encouraged practitioners to use the femoral artery approach on the same side as the kidney that was to be visualized. Although they did not use an image intensifier, they believed it would be beneficial. They considered it important that the injection of contrast medium into a single kidney was not accompanied by the unpleasant burning sensation in the pelvis and legs that was common when injection was made into the aorta for the same purpose.

Their 1956 paper reported successful use of the U-shaped catheter in nine cases and difficulty in only one case. Modestly they concluded the paper by writing, "Because of the continued discussion regard-

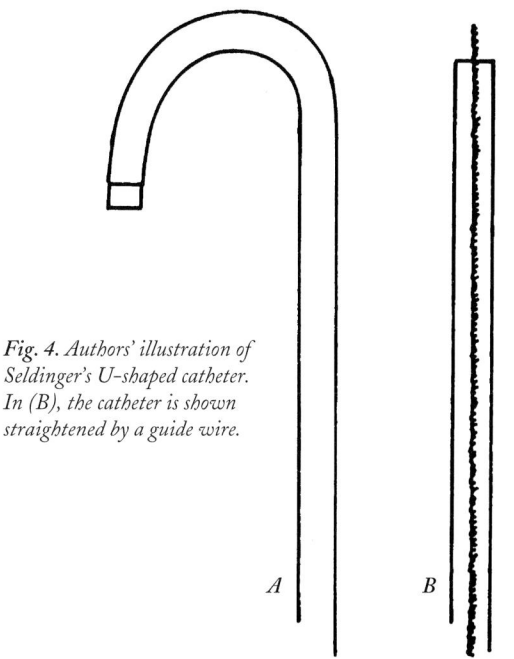

Fig. 4. Authors' illustration of Seldinger's U-shaped catheter. In (B), the catheter is shown straightened by a guide wire.

ing the hazards of aortography, it is too early to judge the roentgenologic value of the method reported. It may, anyhow, be adequate in selected cases where special care of the kidneys is necessary."

During the 1985 interview, Seldinger spoke about the development of the U-shaped catheter. He, like others to follow, fabricated his own equipment, placing an ordinary catheter over a stiff wire and bending both the wire and the catheter into a U shape. The width of the U was about the diameter of the aorta. To soften the catheter, he heated the equipment in steam from a coffeepot. He then plunged the catheter into cold water to stiffen it. When he withdrew the wire, the catheter retained its U shape at the tip.

There is no doubt that Seldinger's two major contributions—percutaneous catheterization and percutaneous introduction of the curved catheter for selective visualization of the renal arteries—changed the way angiography was performed despite the fact that neither contribution was recognized immediately. Both contributions permitted radiologists of ordinary manual dexterity to gain access to vessels, cysts, and hollow organs without the need for surgical cut-down.

About Seldinger

Sven Ivar Seldinger was born in Mora, Sweden (about 180 miles northwest of Stockholm), in 1921, making him only thirty-two years old when he developed his famous technique. His grandfather was the inventor of "practical, useful, and simple things," having devised a machine for making pleats in skirts. It is perhaps from him that Seldinger got his inspiration to keep things simple and functional.

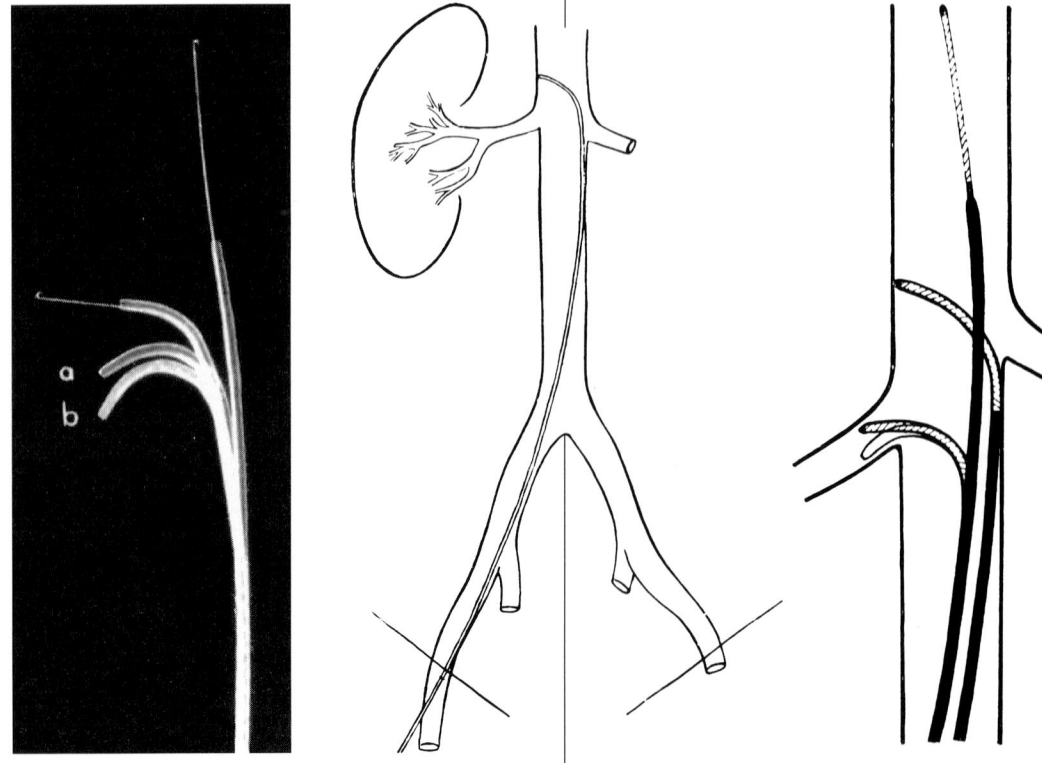

Fig. 5. The U-shaped catheter can be controlled by removing the guide wire (left) and by its placement in the aorta (right).

Seldinger studied medicine at the Karolinska Institute in Stockholm from 1940 to 1948, going back for training in radiology in 1950. After graduation, he stayed on as a staff member until 1966. From 1951 to 1953, he worked on his percutaneous entry technique, and he then applied the technique, using his curved catheter, to visualize renal circulation. Afterwards, he expanded the procedure to visualize other vessels, in particular the thyrocervical artery and the internal mammary artery. In 1966, Seldinger successfully defended his thesis on transhepatic cholangiography, qualifying him as Docent in Radiology the following year.

Soon thereafter, Seldinger returned to his hometown of Mora to continue with his first interest—general radiology. He assumed responsibility for diagnostic radiology at the Lasarett, a rural hospital that he helped build into a state-of-the-art radiological facility.

Seldinger lectured on his research throughout Europe and the United States, and in 1975 he received the Valentine award from the New York Academy of Medicine. A few years later, he received an honorary doctorate from the University of Uppsala in Sweden. He is an honorary member of the Swedish Association of Medical Radiology and the German Roentgen Association.

Seldinger was awarded an honorary membership in the Radiological Society of North America in 1991. In 1992, the Society of Cardiovascular and Interventional Radiology presented him with its Pioneers in Interventional Radiology award.

Seldinger lives with his wife Britt-Lis near Lasarett Hospital in Mora. They have three grown children. Adjacent to their house is a studio where he pursues photography and where Britt-Lis, an artist, enjoys painting and etching.

Seldinger is a private person, and though his name is now well known, few know the man well. We found him to be a delightful person with a keen sense of humor.

The Hotbed of Sweden

The fact that Seldinger pioneered his famous technique in Sweden greatly contributed to that country's reputation as the Mecca of radiology in the late 1950s and throughout the 1960s. Seldinger himself was not an educator of percutaneous catheterization, and no one actually had a fellowship with him. Instead, visiting angiographers from around the world learned the procedure from other Swedes who made names for themselves by publicizing their use of the technique.

There were several institutions in Sweden where radiologists received training, including those in Stockholm, Malmö, Göteborg, and Lund. It was not uncommon in those early days for physicians to go to more than one institution during their stay to gain immediate hands-on experience with the technique and new equipment—learning from teachers who had barely known about the technique much before their students. To be in the inner circle of angiographers in the United States and other countries, therefore, one had to include in a résumé that one had studied in Sweden. (At radiological conferences, it was typical to hear someone say, "When I was in Sweden, we did it this way.")

When radiologists returned home from Sweden, they diagnosed problems using what they had learned there until, in the 1970s, they gradually began to take up the discipline of Dotter and intervention. Throughout those early years, though, Sweden maintained an incredible level of importance in the realm of radiology. The country will always be remembered as the place where percutaneous catheterization began and where Sven Ivar Seldinger forever changed the face of radiology. His work charted a course that was followed by radiologists all over the world.

Perplexity
is the beginning
of knowledge.

Kahlil Gibran

Educator and Inventor

Seldinger's percutaneous entry technique revolutionized medicine. The world turned again to Sweden as Per Ödman made major advances in selective visceral angiography, as Olle Olsson developed selective renal arteriography, as Tord Olin conducted the first fluid-dynamic studies with contrast media flow and pressure, and as Erik Boijsen (Figure 1) applied Ödman's work in pancreatic arteriography to the hepatic arterial bed.

There were other prominent Swedish angiographic instructors as well, but Boijsen was deemed the master educator for the Seldinger technique, and he became quite a drawing card for the University of Lund. Eager students from around the world came to study with him. Those who went to Sweden to study at Karolinska or Malmö made a point to spend some time at Lund just to be with Boijsen.

Students went to Sweden to be challenged, and they knew that while at Lund, there would be at least one instructor who was sure to get them "hooked."

In Search of the Hook-Tail Catheter

By the late 1950s, the golden rule governing the use of a simple end-hole catheter was: Do not inject contrast medium until the catheter tip is away from the vessel or heart wall. Failure to obey this rule usually resulted in a host of potentially dangerous consequences, including catheter dislodgment by recoil, catheter whip, and injection of contrast medium into the vessel or heart wall. Any of these events could result in serious injury to the patient.

A particularly disturbing consequence was that the placement of the catheter tip in the heart could cause arrhythmia. Gidlund and Rodriguez-Alvarez

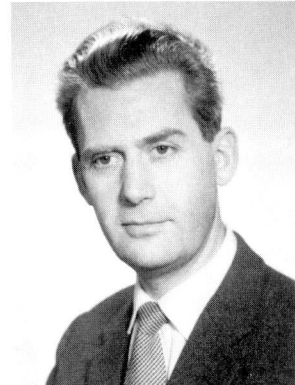

Fig. 1. Erik Boijsen in 1959.

demonstrated in 1956 and 1957 that a closed-end catheter with side holes not only allowed safe, rapid injection of contrast medium but also eliminated recoil. However, to employ the Seldinger percutaneous entry technique, it was desirable to use an open-end catheter.

In 1965, Olin inserted a large bore catheter using the Seldinger technique, then he passed a closed-end catheter with side holes through it. The contrast medium exited the side holes. Other strategies for closing the end hole after percutaneous insertion were described by Tornvall in 1957 and Nordenstrom in 1965. Boijsen provided a simple solution to the problem in 1966: the hook-tail catheter. The end was not completely closed, but its unique fluid-dynamic characteristics made it function almost as if it were. Most important, this curved catheter could be inserted percutaneously with the Seldinger technique.

Creating the Hook-Tail Catheter

Boijsen's hook-tail catheter was made from polyethylene tubing. A wire guide was placed inside, and the distal 3- to 5-cm section was cold-drawn to fit snugly around the guide. Between four and ten side holes were made in the large diameter part

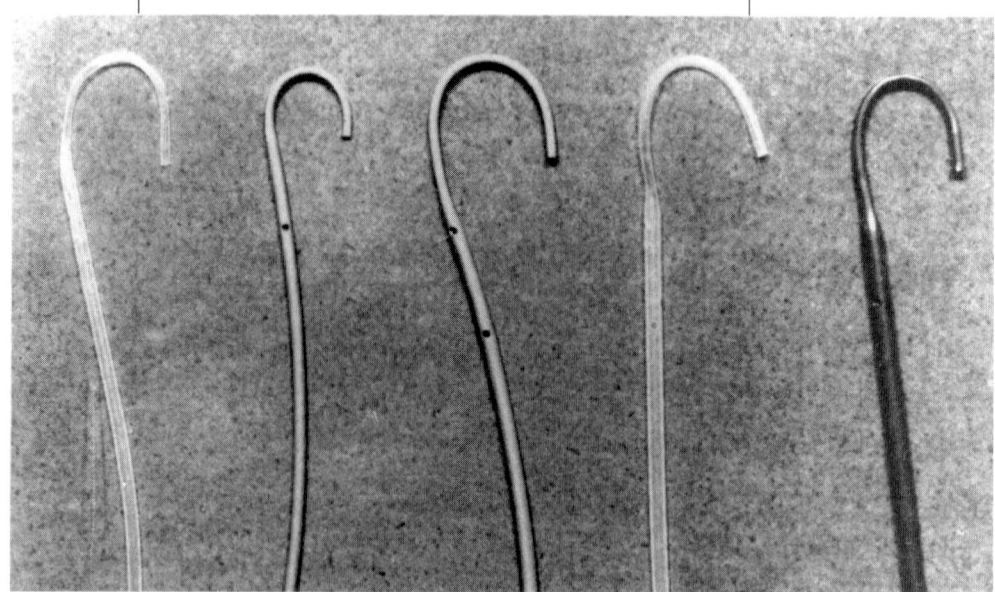

Fig. 2. Boijsen fashioned his hook-tail catheters with a variety of curve sizes.

of the catheter, proximal to the tapered portion.

With the wire guide inside the catheter, Boijsen formed the hook tail by immersing the tapered section of the catheter into hot water and making a 180° bend. The wire guide prevented the curved portion from kinking during the bending process. Boijsen selected the diameter of the hook-tail portion to suit the particular site, such as the aorta or cardiac chambers. When the catheter cooled, he removed the wire guide to restore the original U shape. Figure 2 shows several types of hook-tail catheters with different curve sizes.

Fluid-Dynamic Studies

Boijsen conducted several fluid-dynamic studies using hook-tail catheters and contrast media, availing himself of Olin's expertise and voluminous data from the 1966 studies on flow-pressure characteristics of catheters. He found that the flow/pressure relationships of his hook-tail catheters were almost the same as those of simple open-ended catheters that had no side holes. Further studies revealed that only 10% to 20% of the injected medium flowed out of the small end hole, with the majority leaving by the side holes.

By this time, Boijsen had been joined in Sweden by Charles Dotter's colleague, Melvin Judkins, whom Dotter had sent to study and work with Boijsen. The result of the collaboration was fruitful. There Judkins first saw the Boijsen hook-tail catheter, which Judkins later modified for his left ventriculography angiographic catheters. In their classic 1966 paper on hook-tail catheters for cardioangiography, Boijsen and Judkins reported on two years of experience with 212 patients in whom they studied the right and left heart, aorta, pulmonary artery, and great veins angiographically using percutaneous entry technique.

After this first paper was published, Boijsen used the hook-tail catheter to inject contrast medium into a remarkable variety of vessels. He then published numerous papers on the visualization of the liver and renal circulations, for example.

Fig. 3. Erik Boijsen in his laboratory in 1984.

He also visualized gastric, splenic, and pancreatic vessels, as well as those in the arms and legs. He became adept at selectively injecting contrast medium into very small vessels, including the internal mammary, bronchial, and adrenal cortex arteries.

Smaller and Smaller Vessels

Throughout the years, Boijsen was able to catheterize smaller and smaller vessels in previously inaccessible places; this skill became Boijsen's trademark. He found himself bombarded with invitations to speak throughout the world to angiographers who wanted to hear him describe his techniques so that they too could adopt them.

In commenting on his hook-tail catheter, Boijsen said that it was easy and inexpensive to make and very simple to use. The fluid-dynamic characteristic of the small, flow-resistant tip caused the major portion of the contrast medium to exit the side holes, thus solving the recoil problem and dramatically reducing the risk of wall damage. In addition, the small diameter of the tip allowed wire-guide manipulation of the catheter into small vessels.

Boijsen related that the original name chosen by him and Judkins for their hook-tail catheter was "pigtail" catheter (before Judkins went on to create a pigtail catheter of his own), but the name was changed when a former professor objected to this indelicate term.

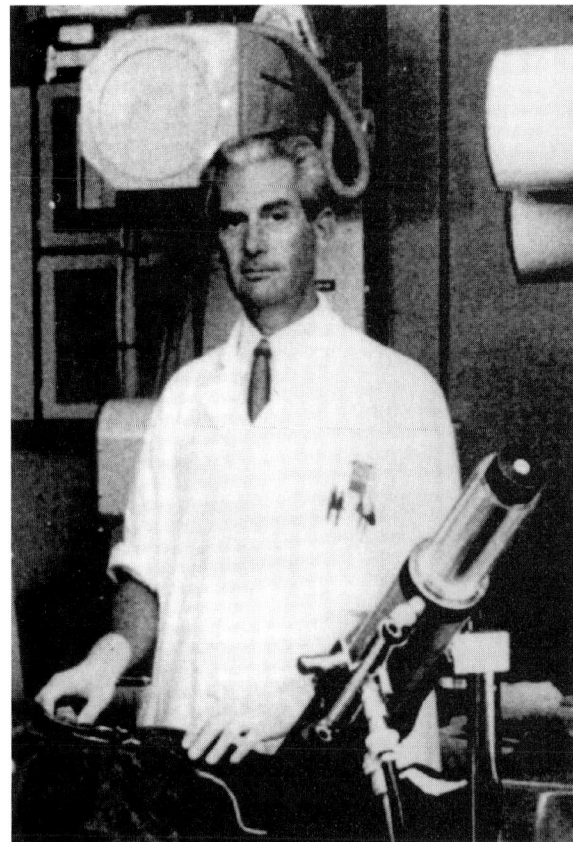

About Boijsen

Erik Boijsen was born to farming parents in Lund, Sweden, in 1922. He stayed in Lund for much of his life, taking premedical courses in high school and entering the University of Lund Medical School after graduating from high school in 1941. Upon graduation from medical school in 1949, he began a residency in Lund, and in 1955 he became a fellow in diagnostic radiology at the University Hospital in Lund and Helsingborg. In 1959, he received a Ph.D. for his angiographic research in renal anatomy. His thesis, "Angiographic Studies of the Anatomy of Single and Multiple Renal Arteries," contains a wealth of beautiful x-rays of the renal vessels.

Boijsen was visiting assistant professor at Stanford University in California during 1962, and subsequently he has been a visiting professor at many other American universities.

From 1970 to 1977, he was professor and chairman of the Department of Radiology at Malmö General Hospital, returning to Lund in 1977 to become professor and chairman of the Department of Radiology at University Hospital. He has published about 150 scientific papers on thoracic, abdominal, and urogenital radiology and has supervised the training of numerous Ph.D. candidates.

AN ACTIVE RETIREMENT

Given his tremendous level of activity throughout his career, it should come as no surprise that Boijsen is leading a very active retirement. He continues his great interest in therapeutic radiology. He serves as editor of *Acta Radiologica*, which is most fortunate since he not only pioneered the field of angiography, but he also has contributed to it over his entire professional life. Even in retirement, Boijsen continues to be in demand.

Loyal to Lund

Despite attractive offers from many countries, Boijsen has remained loyal to Sweden and to Lund, where he built a strong radiology department and continued to conduct clinical research. He is affiliated with several professional associations, is a founder and past president of the European College of Angiography, and is a former vice president of the European Association of Radiologists. Boijsen is an editor, along with three colleagues, for *Frontiers of European Radiology*, and is currently editor-in-chief of *Acta Radiologica*. He is shown in his laboratory in 1984 in Figure 3.

Boijsen lives in Lund with his wife, Maude. They have two children. His daughter is a specialist in radiology at the University of Göteborg. His son is an officer in the Swedish Coast Artillery.

Boijsen Reflects on Radiology Today... and in the Future

In a 1985 interview in Chicago, Boijsen said that his administrative duties were very heavy and he would soon shed them to return to his first love—personal contact with patients and teaching residents and fellows. He said, "We have six sections in diagnostic radiology and everyone is becoming more and more specialized. I have so many good persons in my department who can do specialized radiographic procedures in their subspecialties much better than I can now."

Boijsen indicated he was particularly interested in therapeutic radiology, especially in relation to liver metastasis. He described a procedure in which he injects a chemotherapeutic agent selectively into hepatic vessels, making both arterial and venous injections and occluding the vessels to retain the chemotherapeutic agent for a desired length of time.

Boijsen felt strongly that there was still much to learn about the selective injection of chemotherapeutic agents. He observed, "Because of the conservatism of society's desire for excessive self-protection, progress is hindered. I think we have to reconsider.

"Nobody really knows the outcome of the use of such techniques as surgical removal or embolization.... I have seen tumors of the kidneys which have not changed in size over several years. Normal antibodies of the patient maintain the equilibrium. Possibly in the future, it would be feasible to knock out tumors by selective catheterization and still preserve the rest of the functional tissue. We may get other agents, like monoclonal antibodies, which are on their way.

"If we find a carcinoma, we may or may not take it out. With surgery, what we are doing, really, is spreading the cells. If we go in and touch the tumor, many cells leave the tumor. Let it be in peace and treat it like it is! But many surgeons cannot do that. Some are uneasy and when they find a tumor they have to remove it. I think there is some logic here; however, in the last twenty years there has been no improvement in prognosis of most cancers. We must do something else.

"I have seen successful therapy with alcohol injection.... I have seen a remarkable case. There was a patient who had a very large renal carcinoma. I embolized it and the tumor shrank dramatically. After a few months the patient said, 'I feel wonderful. I feel fine. My hair has grown back. I feel perfect now!' The tumor was gone, but later she got a colon carcinoma. However, look at the time that was bought!"

Treating Liver Metastases

Speaking about the therapeutic aspects of interventional radiology, Boijsen said, "I think the most interesting circulation today is the liver's. We should be able to treat metastases of the liver and even to make lobar resection without surgery. We have made preliminary experimental studies by injecting alcohol into hepatic arteries. If injected into the arterial side, it will destroy the vessels. It is dispersed all the way out to the capillary level, which means you can destroy the tumor. But you will also destroy the normal parenchyma. Very little [60%] alcohol is needed, which causes the circulation to close down completely. This method can be used to treat any tumor without surgery.

"The surgeons operate because they believe the tumor should be removed. Nobody has really proved that. Perhaps it is much better to reduce the tumor slowly, so that the body's antibodies can take care of it. I believe that we will be able to destroy the tumor slowly by immunization and then the metastases can be treated as well. Basically, the technique involves merely the selective injection of alcohol into the tumor. The procedure is repeated several times because the body has a tremendous capacity to compete with whatever you are doing."

Many physicians from around the world have come to the University of Lund for specialized training in diagnostic radiology. Boijsen seems to know them all. Among the Americans were Melvin Judkins, Herbert Abrams, Robert Mosely, Mark Wholey, Sidney Wallace, Stewart Reuter, and Helen Redman. Each turned to Boijsen as they learned the Seldinger technique, for he was the undisputed master. Even in his retirement, Boijsen continues to confront the challenges of therapeutic radiology as he seeks new ways to attack age-old diseases.

Art is I;

science is we.

Claude Bernard

Inventing Tapered, Flexible-Tip Catheters

Sometimes a researcher spends years trying to find a solution to a problem and never succeeds. At other times, a solution just falls into the lap of someone not even looking for it. It takes a perceptive researcher to realize the significance of such a serendipitous discovery and to publicize it so that others may be enlightened.

In the 1950s, Mason Sones, Jr., (Figure 1) was a pediatric cardiologist at the Cleveland Clinic. One day, he placed a catheter into what he thought was the patient's left ventricle and made a high-pressure injection. To his dismay, the catheter was actually in a coronary artery. Until that time, physicians had avoided placing catheters into coronary arteries, fearing the procedure would cause arrhythmia or block blood supply in the artery and result in a heart attack. Fortunately, that was not the case with Sones' patient. In fact, Sones had accidentally discovered that he could inject into coronary arteries and obtain good pictures. Hence he made one of the greatest discoveries in the history of angiography and became the father of selective coronary arteriography.

Sones showed the world of radiology that with an appropriately designed catheter and good manipulative technique, one could selectively catheterize human coronary arteries and make those arteries visible by injecting only a few milliliters of contrast medium using simple manual force applied to the injection syringe. Before this, a large volume of contrast medium was injected rapidly into the aortic root under high pressure to secure coronary opacification. Even with this method, the coronary arteries were not always visualized clearly, a circumstance that inspired Sones to pioneer the use of an image intensifier in combination with high-speed photography.

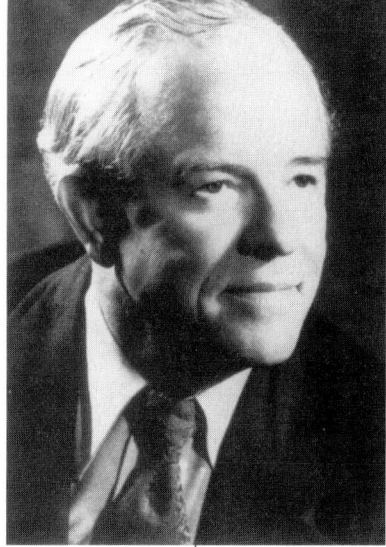

Fig. 1. Mason Sones, 1918-1985.

Sones' discoveries formed the background to selective coronary catheterization, which began in 1956—the year that Sones developed a catheter with assistance from United States Catheter and Instrument Company (USCI).

The Quest for Better Images

Sones had a keen desire to improve the quality of angiograms. He had heard of the image intensifier and decided to spend one week in Russell Morgan's laboratory at Johns Hopkins. Morgan was the authority on the device. When Sones recognized that the equipment was essential for coronary angiography, he obtained a 5-inch unit from the Phillips Company of Holland and started to experiment. In 1956, he initiated a series of tests in dogs using the device to view coronary arteries. Although he was able to view both normal and surgically ligated coronary arteries with the intensifier, he realized a larger unit would be necessary for human studies.

Working with Phillips Company engineers, Sones helped develop an 11-inch image intensifier equipped with a Schmidt optical system and a 35-mm movie camera. The device was placed in operation in 1958 for clinical trials at the Cleveland Clinic. In a series of fifty patients without coronary disease, the main coronary arteries could be visualized in only thirty-four patients. Secondary and tertiary vessels could rarely be identified. The contrast medium produced an uncomfortable sense of heat that was accompanied by peripheral flush—symptoms not tolerated well by patients.

From this study, it became apparent that the geometric relationship between the viewing screen of the 11-inch intensifier and the 35-mm motion picture film was not right for detailed visualization of the coronary arteries. Furthermore, the 11-inch intensifier was susceptible to scattered x-rays. A smaller x-ray field was needed for high-resolution imaging; the 5-inch intensifier would be satisfactory for that purpose.

Sones' 11-inch image intensifier was not used for very long, but it played an important role in bringing about selective coronary arteriography. Figure 2 shows Sones' laboratory with the six-foot-long, 11-inch image intensifier mounted below an x-ray table with the x-ray tube placed above. A pit had to be built into the floor so that the intensified image could be viewed. The input phosphor (under the table) had to face upward because of design limitations. To view the intensified image, Sones climbed into the pit and looked up at the output phosphor (Figure 3). Therefore, to perform a coronary angiogram, one operator had to be with the patient on the table to inject the contrast medium while another operator was below the table, viewing and photographing the image.

A Revolutionary Discovery

On October 30, 1958, Sones made a revolutionary discovery. During a routine left ventricular imaging study, Sones (from the submerged pit)

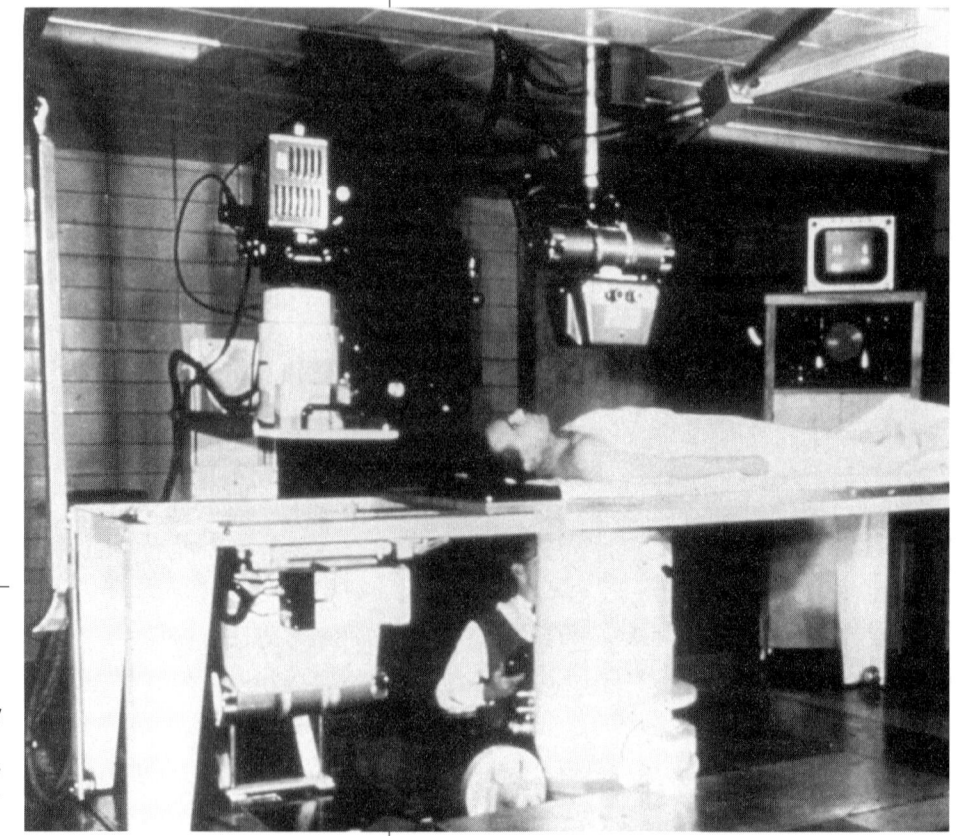

Fig. 2. This is the cardiac laboratory devised by Sones in the 1950s. Shown are the 11-inch image intensifier placed below the table and the x-ray tube placed above the patient, who is on a radiolucent table.

requested that the catheter tip be withdrawn to just above the aortic valve so that contrast medium could be injected into the sinus of Valsalva. Describing the event, Sones wrote:

> My associate, Dr. Royston Lewis, made an injection of 40 cc of 90% Hypaque through the catheter. About one second before the injection was initiated, I hit the switch to initiate a cine run.
>
> When the injection began, I was horrified to see the right coronary artery become heavily opacified and realized the catheter tip was actually inside the orifice of the dominant right coronary artery. I shouted, 'Pull it out!' Our combined reaction times to accomplish withdrawal of the catheter consumed from three to four seconds, which meant that approximately 30 cc of 90% Hypaque had been delivered into the right coronary artery. I was of course horrified because I was certain that the patient would develop ventricular fibrillation. At that time we did not have direct current defibrillators and knew nothing about the application of closed chest cardiac massage.
>
> I climbed out of the hole and ran around the table looking for a scalpel to open his chest in order to defibrillate him by direct application of the paddles of an alternating current defibrillator. I looked at the oscilloscope tracing of his electrocardiogram and it was evident that he was in asystole rather than ventricular fibrillation. I knew that an explosive cough could produce a very effective pressure pulse in the aorta and hoped this might push the contrast media through his myocardial capillary bed. Fortunately, he was still conscious and responded to my demand that he cough repeatedly. After three or four explosive coughs, his heart began to beat again with initially a sinus bradycardia which accelerated to sinus tachycardia within 15 to 20 seconds. He then made a perfectly uneventful recovery with no neurological deficit or other sequelae.
>
> Initially, I could feel only unbelievable relief and gratitude that we had been fortunate enough to avert a grievous disaster. During the ensuing days I began to think that this accident might point the way for the development of a technique which was exactly what we had been seeking. If a human could tolerate such a massive injection of contrast media directly into a coronary artery, it might be possible to accomplish this type of an opacification with small doses of more dilute contrast agent. With considerable fear and trepidation, we embarked on a program to accomplish this objective.

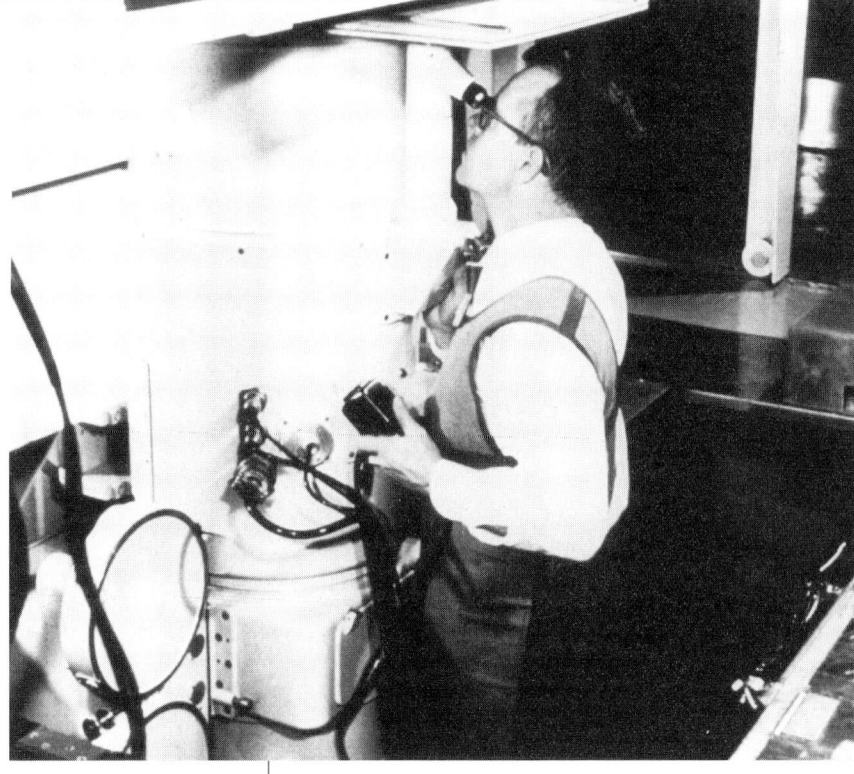

Fig. 3. Here is Mason Sones in the pit looking up at an intensified image on his 11-inch intensifier.

The Flexible Catheter

Sones used the left brachial artery approach to the coronary arteries. A description of his special-purpose catheter, fabricated by USCI and delivered in April of 1959, appeared in *Modern Concepts of Cardiovascular Disease* in 1962. It read, "The shaft of this thin-walled radiopaque woven catheter is 2.7 mm in external diameter (8 French) to provide enough rigidity for dependable manipulations in the systolic jet immediately and above the aortic valve. The tip is open and four openings are arranged in opposite pairs within 7 mm of its distal end. The shaft is sharply tapered to an external diameter of 1.6 mm (5 French) at a point 5 cm from its tip. This provides an extremely flexible 'finger tip' which may be curved upward into the coronary orifices by pressure of the more rigid

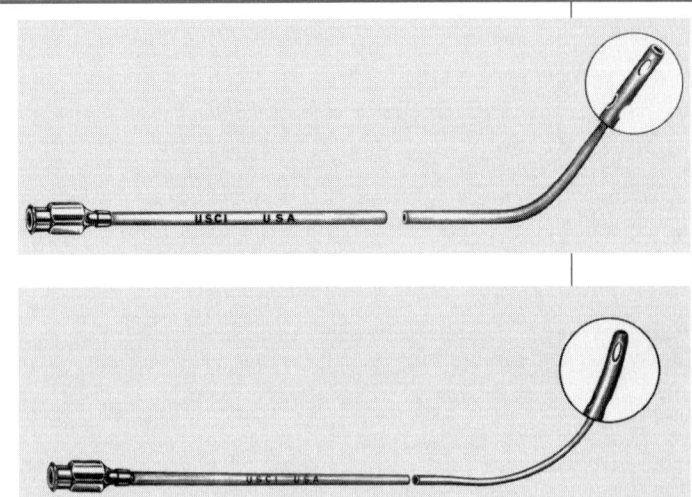

Fig. 4. The Sones flexible-tip catheters from a USCI catalog.

shaft against the aortic valve cusps. This maneuver is demonstrated in the motion picture previously described. It has been possible to enter both coronary arteries in 954 of 1,020 patients studied. In no instance has failure to enter at least one vessel occurred. Since each artery is routinely photographed in multiple projections, a total of 7,207 individual arteriograms were recorded in this group of patients."

Sones' flexible-tip catheter is shown in Figure 4. Figure 5 shows the catheter advancing toward the left and right coronary ostia.

First Mention

Sones first mentioned his new selective catheter in Chapter 8 of the book *Clinical Cardiopulmonary Physiology*, which was published in 1960. In commenting on the results of a two-hundred-patient study, he wrote, "The slow manual injection of from 3 cc to a maximum of 6 cc of contrast media by this technique provides uniformly dependable visualization of either vessel.... As many as six serial injections of contrast media have been made into each coronary artery orifice at one to three minute intervals using the media and doses described above, without evidence of myocardial injury. In no instance has perfusion with the media resulted in the development of abdominal pain, electrocardiographic ischemia, or photographic evidence of coronary artery constrictions....

"With very heavy coronary opacification, transient depression or elevation of the T-wave in the electrocardiogram occurs at the moment when the media is in maximum concentration in the arterioles and capillary bed of the myocardium. This is accompanied by bradycardia. A gradual return of the T-waves and heart rate to the pre-injection state occurs during the following 10 to 20 seconds. This may be accelerated by asking the patient to take one or two deep breaths."

It was not until 1962 that Sones felt confident enough to describe his clinical results. Characteristically, he waited until he had performed coronary angiograms successfully on one thousand patients. The paper appeared in Volume 31 of *Modern Concepts in Cardiovascular Disease* in 1962 and was only four pages long.

Identifying Small Vessels

In his next paper, published in July 1962, Sones reported the use of his technique in 2,500 coronary artery visualizations. The angiograms allowed identification of coronary vessels as small as 100 to 200 microns. By 1967, Sones reported that he and his colleagues had performed coronary arteriograms on 8,200 patients, representing all types of atherosclerosis. In more than 99% of the cases, both coronary arteries could be visualized.

Although Sones' catheter was modified by many (by adding curves and metal braid), the original version had some unique features. For example, the same catheter could be used for visualizing the aorta, the left ventricle, and both coronary arteries. Its flexible tip, when advanced against the aortic valves, permitted the creation of a loop that facilitated entry into the coronary ostia. Perhaps most important, angiographers of ordinary skill could easily master its use.

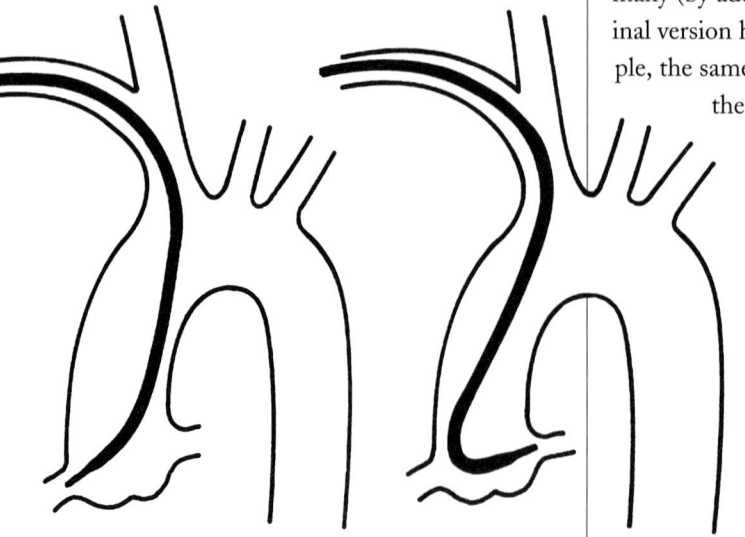

Fig. 5. Illustration shows the Sones flexible-tip catheter entering the right and left coronary arteries.

Interestingly, Sones never performed a Seldinger percutaneous entry procedure and continued to use the cut-down technique even after the Seldinger method was popularized.

About Sones

Mason Sones was born on October 28, 1918, in Noxapater, Mississippi. His father was a machinist and his mother a homemaker. Sones attended high school in Baltimore and was active in photography and swimming. He attended Western Maryland College in Westminster, Maryland, received the B.A. degree, and was drum major of the school band. In 1942, he married Geraldine Newton. They had three sons and one daughter.

Sones received his M.D. degree from the University of Maryland School of Medicine in 1943 and spent one year there as an intern. He then served in the United States Air Force from 1944 to 1946 in the Pacific, after which he entered a residency program in internal medicine at the Henry Ford Hospital in Detroit. After completing this program in 1950, he became director of pediatric cardiology and of the cardiac laboratory at the Cleveland Clinic Foundation, a position he held until 1975, when he became senior physician in the Department of Cardiology.

An Influential Innovator

As a pediatric cardiologist, Sones was one of the first to use cardiac catheterization in neonates. He also constantly strove to perfect radiographic techniques, being among the earliest to apply the motion-picture camera to an image-intensifier tube and to use a television camera (Dage vidicon) to display real-time x-ray images on a television monitor.

The Cleveland Clinic was quick to use the many high-quality diagnostic angiographic techniques developed by Sones, and physicians came from all over to learn the Sones technique of selective coronary arteriography. One of them was Melvin Judkins, who took the Sones method to the University of Oregon. He found that the Sones catheter did not perform well in patients with a dilated aorta. To solve this problem he developed his own selective catheters.

In the spring of 1978, USCI launched a new product, the woven-sleeve catheter. It provided improved torque control for the Sones catheter and later became available with curved tips to accommodate easy entry into the left and right coronary orifices in patients with varying aortic shapes. To commemorate a twenty-one year association with Sones and to recognize the contributions of their employees in developing the woven catheter, USCI held an appreciation day on May 25, 1978, at its Glens Falls, New York, plant. On that occasion Sones was taken up in a hot-air balloon (Figure 6) while employees and guests cheered.

Mason Sones was not a prolific writer. His curriculum vitae lists sixty-six publications, of

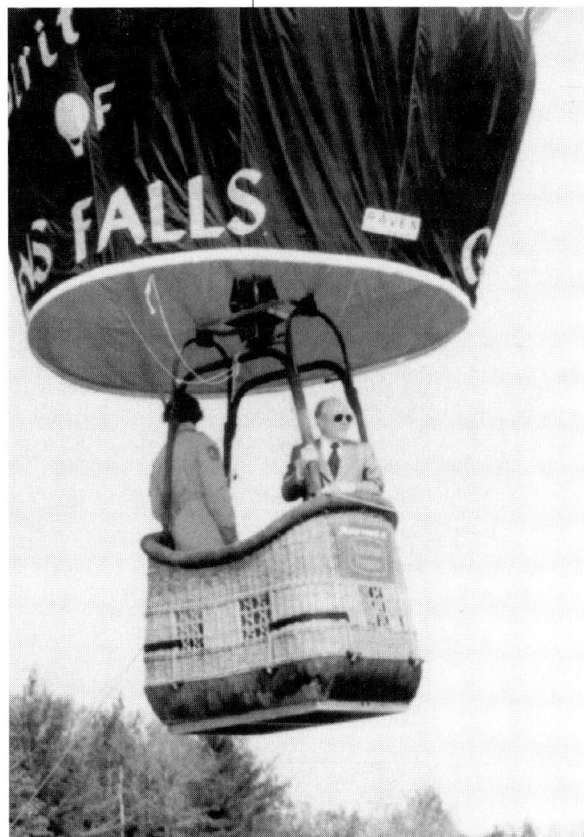

Fig. 6. *On May 25, 1978, Mason Sones was carried aloft by balloon to commemorate 21 years of close association with USCI. (Courtesy of USCI)*

SIGNIFICANT ACHIEVEMENTS

Through Sones' work, the volume of contrast medium required for coronary visualization was reduced tenfold over the aortic root injection technique and only manual pressure was required for injection. The success rate in coronary imaging was soon to increase to above 99% and the risk to the myocardium was minimal. The unpleasant peripheral heat and flush sensations experienced by patients who underwent coronary angiography prior to the Sones technique were reduced.

which he is the senior author on only eighteen. Perhaps this is consistent with his view of himself as a team player. Although a rugged individualist, Sones truly believed that the team approach was the only way to provide the best care for his patients. His secretary, Beverly Cohn, recalled his response to her inquiry about her job: "You don't work for me; we are a team."

Forceful Personality

All who knew Mason Sones were aware of his forceful personality. Irvine Page wrote, "I knew [him as] a small, chubby, bumptious man who worked incessantly and swore with gusto." Perhaps his dominant characteristic was a missionary-like striving for perfection, accuracy, and truth. Fred Schoonmaker said that Sones' frequent comment about his own work was, "It's not good enough."

Sones' zeal for accuracy could manifest itself in open disagreement with a lecturer making a scientific presentation at a conference. Although some thought this behavior to be overbearing and perhaps arrogant, his disagreement was usually justified by his pointing out that the speaker had overlooked evidence that was obvious from data presented in the speaker's own support material.

One particularly memorable episode happened at an annual scientific meeting of the American Heart Association. A guest speaker was showing a slide and uttered the words, "In this normal coronary arteriogram . . ." Before he could get another word out, Sones stood up in the back of the room and said, "That's not normal! There's a stenosis in one of the coronary arteries!" Sones was correct. Though not intentionally trying to embarrass anyone, Sones' relentless quest for truth and accuracy caused more than one public speaker to suffer some indignity.

In his working years, Sones had no time for hobbies, stating that his vocation was his avocation. In his final years, he did have the opportunity to play golf, fish, and travel. He had a childlike wonder for nature's beauty and took a video camera on many trips to preserve beauty as he saw it. On August 29, 1985, Mason Sones died of lung cancer at the age of sixty-six.

Sones' Many Honors

The Sones technique became accepted because of the overwhelming results it produced. This acceptance is evidenced by Sones' many honors and awards from scientific societies. One of the first was the Golden Eagle Award for cinematography, which was conferred on him three times—in 1963, 1966, and 1969. The American College of Chest Physicians presented him with its Film Award in 1963. The American Medical Association honored him with its Film Award in 1966 and the Scientific Achievement Award in 1976. In 1979, he received a gold medal from the Radiological Society of North America. The American College of Cardiology recognized his contributions by awarding him its Presidential Citation.

Sones also received honors from numerous foreign countries. The Royal College of Physicians (London) invited him to present the Haile Selassie Lecture, and the Worshipful Society of Apothecaries of London awarded him the prestigious Galen Medal in 1985. Argentina's Federal University of LaPlata awarded him a doctorate, honoris causa. The Favaloro Foundation of Buenos Aires awarded him a gold medal, and the Brazilian Air Force in 1982 presented him its Order of Merit. The same award was also presented by the State of São Paulo, Brazil, and the Brazilian government conferred upon him the Presidential Order of Merit.

Sones received an honorary doctorate from Western Maryland College in 1968, and his alma mater, the University of Maryland, named him Alumnus of the Year in 1969. The journal *Modern Medicine* presented its Distinguished Achievement Award to him in 1966, the same year he received the Theodore and Susan Cummings Humanitarian Award. Among the other awards Sones received were the Gaindner Foundation International Award (1969) and the Roy C. Fish Award from the Texas Heart Institute. In 1981, the journal *Medical Times* presented him the Physician of Excellence Award, and in 1963 he received the Albert Lasker Clinical Medicine Research Award.

Sones was a fellow in six professional societies, including the American College of Cardiology, the American College of Chest Physicians, and the Society for Cardiac Angiography. He was an honorary fellow in eight scientific societies, including the American College of Radiology, and was a member of six other professional organizations.

Great things are not done by those of faint heart. To achieve great things takes a special personality and tenacity. What Mason Sones accomplished led to even greater breakthroughs. His serendipitous accident led to the development of selective coronary arteriography. Without coronary arteriography it would be impossible to select patients for coronary arterial bypass and angioplasty.

Although most accidents are associated with misfortune, Sones' discovery was certainly the result of very good luck—for him and for countless patients.

Ah, to build,
to build!
That is the noblest
of all the arts.

Henry Wadsworth Longfellow

CHAPTER 5: Melvin P. Judkins

Approaching the Heart from a Different Angle

"When you wake up, get up. When you get up, do something." This simple maxim, a favorite of Melvin Judkins (Figure 1), tells you a lot about the man and predicts his commitment to finding a better way.

Judkins developed catheters that enable selective injection of contrast medium into the right and left coronary arteries and the technique that uses these catheters. Judkins was familiar with catheters from his early training as a urologist. Later training in general radiology and a familiarity with the Seldinger percutaneous entry technique led him in 1967 to develop an alternative to the Sones cut-down method for coronary artery catheterization. He became one of the best of a rare breed from the early days of percutaneous catheterization—a radiologist who specialized in coronary arteriography.

A Percutaneous Method
Sones' brachial artery cut-down technique worked effectively, but Judkins saw problems with it when applied to patients in whom the aorta was dilated. In the Sones technique, the inserted catheter was guided to a coronary artery orifice by the curvature of the aorta. However, when the aorta was dilated, guidance was uncertain. Judkins set out to develop a simpler and more reliable method that could be applied to both the dilated and the normal aorta.

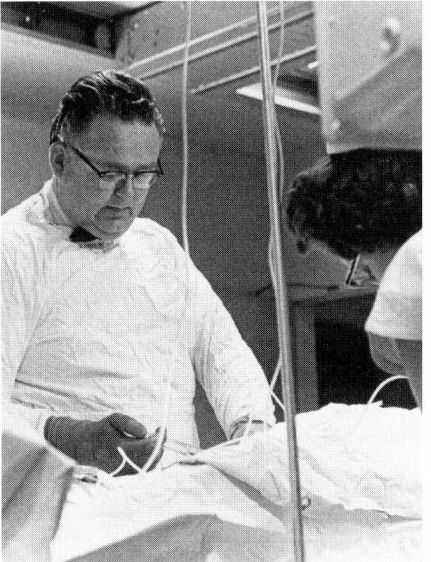

Judkins maintained that the success of his method was due to the combination of special catheters for the left and right coronary arteries and the technique in which these catheters were used. Technical highlights of the Judkins procedure included the percutaneous transfemoral approach and use of coronary-seeking catheters of his own

Fig. 1. Melvin Judkins in 1968.

design. The coronary-seeking catheters greatly simplified selective coronary arteriography and increased the ease and confidence with which angiographers could place catheters. Judkins himself commented in 1985, "The catheters know where to go if not thwarted by the operator!"

Although Judkins used his femoral artery technique almost exclusively, rather than Sones' brachial artery method, he did not claim superiority of his own technique over the other. He did, however, advocate that an angiographer select one approach and become proficient in it, stating in 1974, "The two techniques are as different as day and night; the finger calisthenics required for their performance are entirely different."

The Shape of Things to Come

Before the availability of preformed angiographic catheters, Judkins shaped Cordis catheters at the time of each examination, as he had done in Sweden. He placed polyurethane tubing over a stiff wire bent to conform to the shape of the

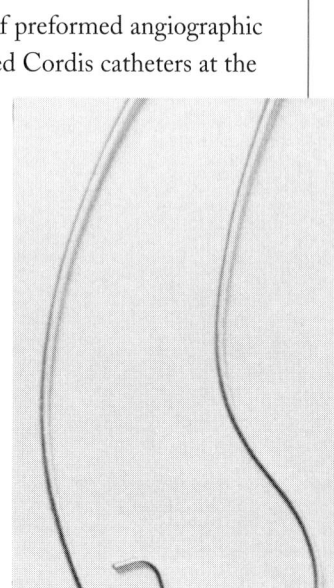

Fig. 2. These left and right coronary catheters developed by Judkins have tips that are 5.5 French and have an I.D. of 0.041 in. The body is 8 French with an I.D. of 0.056 in. A 12-strand braid of stainless steel wire is incorporated into its wall. The braid ensures good torque control.

vessel, and then he immersed the catheter in boiling water to soften it. When the assembly cooled, he withdrew the wire, and the catheter retained its shape.

The right and left coronary artery catheters designed by Judkins (Figure 2) had three bends. The angles and the length of catheter tubing between bends were distinctly different in the left and right coronary catheters.

Judkins introduced the catheter through the femoral artery. When it reached the region of the aortic arch and the ascending aorta, he removed the wire guide, manipulated the preformed curves along the wall of

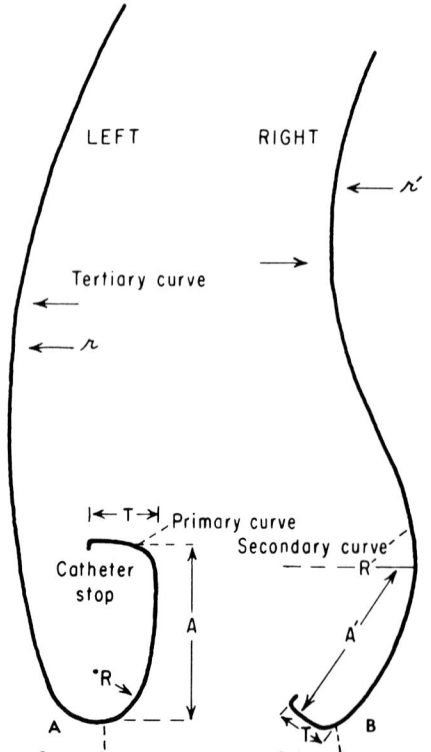

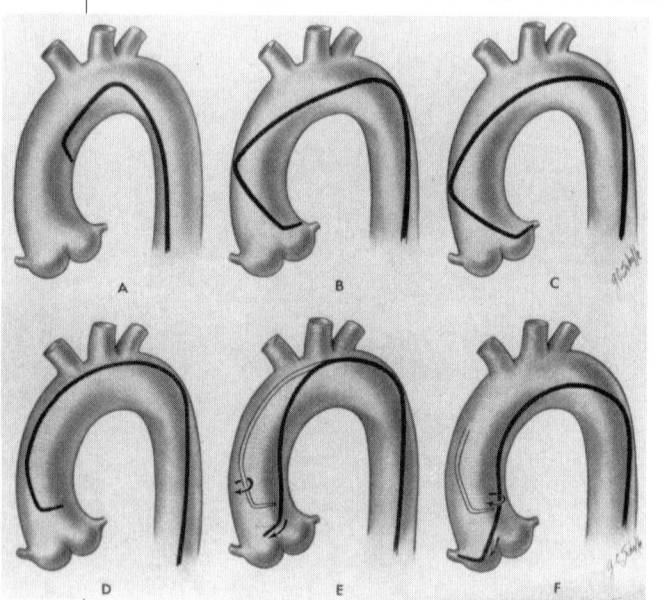

Fig. 3. In Judkins' coronary catheter technique, the guide is removed as the catheter is advanced through the proximal descending thoracic aorta. (A) through (C) show placement in the left coronary artery; (D) through (F) in the right.

the aortic arch, and positioned the catheter to enter the appropriate ostium (Figure 3). The relative ease of the percutaneous transfemoral approach and the predictability of placement of the catheter tip into a coronary ostium were the reasons for the popularity of the Judkins technique and its worldwide acceptance.

According to Robert C. Stevens (formerly with Cordis Corporation), in 1967 Judkins heat-formed the Cordis polyurethane catheter with braided steel wire in the wall. Stevens had developed the steel-braid-reinforced Ducor catheter to withstand high-pressure injection and to impart rotational control. Because a wire guide did not pass easily into the tip of the polyurethane catheter, Judkins sought help from Bill Cook

(Cook Incorporated), who provided Teflon-coated safety wire guides that passed smoothly through the tip. Manufacture of Judkins' curved polyurethane catheters was taken up by Cordis Corporation in 1968.

Different Shapes

In 1962, Ricketts and Abrams had reported the percutaneous insertion of catheters, preformed to the anatomy of the aortic arch, into the coronary arteries of dogs and later into patients, via a femoral artery. The shapes of their two catheters, designed for entry into the coronaries, were such that the tip was directed to the target ostium by guidance from the aortic wall. As Judkins would later recognize, and Ricketts and Abrams observed, "The simple expedient of developing two catheters of different shape, each molded so as to enter the ostia of one or the other coronary artery, permitted rapid and reliable insertion of the catheter tip into the appropriate orifice."

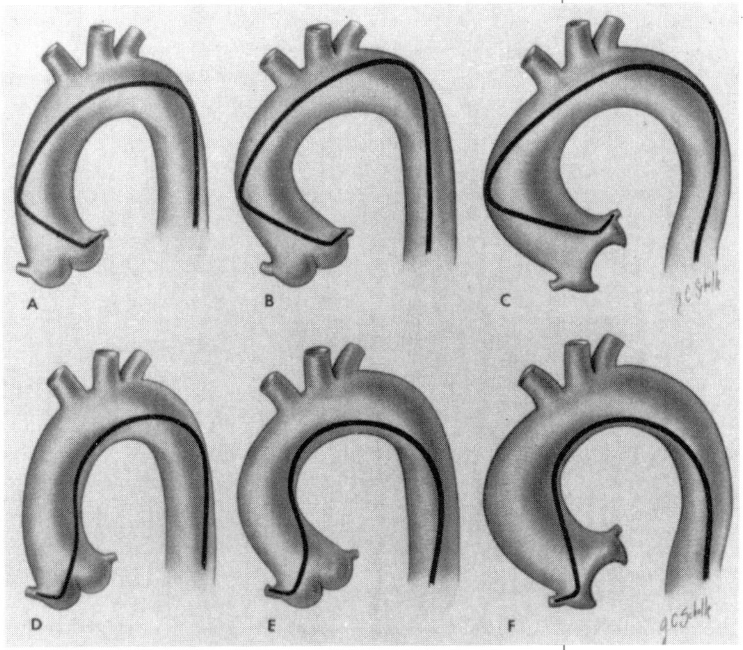

Many of Judkins' early selective cardioangiographic studies were conducted on patients with aortic valve disease and postvalvular enlargement of the aorta. Other types of cardiovascular disease, the patient's age, and individual anatomic variations led Judkins in 1968 to identify at least three types of aortic configurations: normal, unfolded, and poststenotic. To accommodate the various sizes and shapes of aortic roots, catheter dimensions were modified appropriately. Small, medium, and large catheters were fashioned in which the distances between individual bends in the catheter and the radii of curvature differed (Figure 4).

Two innovations during the 1960s enhanced the ability of physicians to negotiate tortuous or atherosclerotic vessels. In these vessels, stiff, straight wire guides and catheters posed the threats of damaging the vessel wall or of breaking within the vessel, allowing pieces to become separated and lost in the circulatory system.

These difficulties in catheterizing tortuous vessels led to the 1964 Baum and Abrams use of a J-shaped catheter, whose rounded distal tip more easily negotiated the sharp bends and luminal discontinuities presented by atheromatous plaque. The J-shaped catheters were followed by flexible wire guides shaped with a bend at the tip. Still, however, the possibility of wire guide breakage within the vessel was real; any sharp bending of the wire guide weakened the instrument, and the stresses encountered with repeated manipulations through tortuous vessels increased the chance of breakage. Publication (by Dotter, Judkins, and Frische in 1966 and Judkins, Kidd, Frische, and Dotter in 1967) of the use of the Cook Safe-T-J wire guide, however, established this innovation as a solution to the problem.

In 1967, Judkins recommended that if resistance to passage of a standard wire guide was encountered in the iliofemoral vessel, the wire guide should be removed and replaced with a Teflon-coated Safe-T-J guide. If resistance continued to be met and the Safe-T-J guide could not be advanced after a brief manipulation, Judkins advised that one should "forget it" and try another vessel.

Fig. 4. Judkins' technique allowed for differences in sizes and shapes of aortic roots: small (A, D), medium (B, E), and large (C, F). Note the distances between catheter bends.

THE SAFE-T-J GUIDE WIRE

The Cook Safe-T-J guide was a flexible wire coil with a tapered metal mandrel that provided stiffness at its core. The mandrel was shorter than the coil guide, and its tapered distal tip permitted a lesser degree of stiffness near the guide's distal tip. Within the core was a fine safety wire, soldered to both ends of the coil. In the event of wire-guide breakage, this safety wire kept any broken pieces from becoming separated from the rest of the guide. Furthermore, the guide's design enabled the distal tip to be curved into a J-shape.

Paying Attention to Details

In the late 1960s, coronary angiography was performed by many physicians, but Judkins' name was prominent in the field. Published papers do not reveal the entire reason; however, a 1986 personal communication to the authors from Stevens provides the critical information. Stevens wrote, "In late 1967, Judkins telephoned me to say that he had shaped my Ducor catheter into the perfect left and right coronary catheters. I flew to Portland to visit him and watched him as he and his team performed three coronary studies, back to back, in less than two hours! Total turn-around time for the studies themselves averaged fifteen minutes!"

Judkins considered an examination of the coronary arteries incomplete without ventriculography to assess ventricular function. Problems associated with injecting contrast medium into the ventricular cavity through a straight catheter with a single end port had been previously recognized. The 1966 Boijsen-Judkins hook-tail catheter with multiple side holes reduced many of these problems.

The Pigtail Catheter

Judkins went on to introduce the pigtail catheter for ventriculographic studies. The catheter incorporated an elongated, coiled tip and multiple side holes located proximal to the tapered terminal segment (Figure 5). Multiple side ports accommodated rapid injection of contrast medium without the damaging effect of a jet from a single end port directed against the endocardium. The coiled design helped stabilize the catheter during injection of contrast medium and prevented it from whipping within the ventricular cavity and digging into tissue. As if to emphasize appropriateness of the design for minimizing endocardial trauma, Judkins wrote in 1968, "Even the most 'ham-handed' of operators will find it difficult to obtain a subendocardial injection with this catheter."

Blood-pressure monitoring was routine in Judkins' laboratory. He advised in 1968, "Careful, constant catheter tip pressure is essential! If there is any damping of pressure or slowed washout on test injection, the catheter should be removed and repositioned."

Complication Rate

A 1973 report in *Circulation* by Adams, Fraser, and Abrams apparently touched a raw nerve in Judkins. The report presented

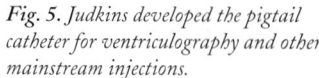

Fig. 5. Judkins developed the pigtail catheter for ventriculography and other mainstream injections.

results of a survey that inquired about the incidence of various complications associated with coronary arteriography. The responses revealed a significantly higher complication rate with the Judkins transfemoral technique than with the Sones brachial artery method. The study also indicated that the complication rate decreased as the number of selective coronary angiograms at a given institution increased.

One can sense Judkins' irritation when he (with Gander) referred to the survey report in a *Circulation* editorial the following year. The editorial stated, "There is no question that the femoral technique's ease of performance and quality of examination induces many to undertake it with scarcely any grounding, most with no apparent sense of their inadequacies. Such misadventure can be expected to generate a high percentage of complications."

Judkins stated that not only was the "complication rate inversely related to the number of procedures performed annually in a given laboratory, but as the number of examinations increases . . . the complication disparity between the brachial and the femoral approach dramatically narrows to near equality."

As a pioneer in coronary angiography, Melvin Judkins never lost sight of the fact that the success of the technique credited to him was due to the careful combination of many elements, each requiring meticulous attention. While he will be remembered as more than just a designer of angiographic catheters, that accomplishment alone is enough to secure his place in history.

About Judkins

Melvin Judkins was born in 1922 in Los Angeles, California. Health service ran deep through his family; his father was a physical therapist, two uncles were physicians, and several aunts were nurses. As a boy he was interested in all things mechanical and electrical, being fond of making crystal sets in the early days of radio. He enjoyed playing with model trains and loved building things. An aptitude test revealed that he would do well in engineering or medicine, and for a time he favored making a career of engineering.

In 1940, he enrolled in the premedical program at La Sierra College (now Loma Linda University), where he received a B.S. degree in 1945. His favorite college subject was physics. He then enrolled in Loma Linda Medical School, his education supported by the U.S. Army. While in medical school, he met Eileen Cobb and married her one week before they both graduated in 1947—she as a nurse and he as a physician. After graduation, he interned for one year at Loma Linda Hospital.

In 1947, Judkins fulfilled his military obligation with a two-year tour of duty that led to his achieving the rank of captain and becoming chief of the urology section at the 28th General Hospital of the U.S. Army in Osaka, Japan. During this preradiology period of his career, Judkins published a paper in a 1949 edition of the *Far East Army Medical Journal* on a new surgical technique for varicocele. It was from these days in urology that Judkins gained experience with catheters.

After leaving the Army, Judkins enrolled in a residency program (1949–1950) at the University of California Medical Center in Sacramento. Following his residency, he was engaged in general medical practice until 1960. For about the first year, he worked in Sumas, Washington, twenty miles from the Pacific coast and the Canadian border. The isolation of the town—with the nearest hospital twenty-five miles away, heavy snowfall, and persistent night calls—led him to seek employment in a different location. He settled down in Antioch, California, a small manufacturing town near San Francisco. This practice provided broad experience with industrial accident cases.

Interest in Radiology

The need to have x-ray films read by a radiologist stimulated Judkins' interest in radiology. He applied to several residency programs, including one at the Mayo Clinic and another at the University of Oregon. The Mayo Clinic turned him down because of his age, but the University of Oregon accepted him.

After a brief vacation in Europe before beginning his residency, Judkins returned to the University of Oregon, where he came under the influence and guidance of Charles Dotter. It was here that Albert Starr was implanting his well-known Starr-Edwards prosthetic valve. Starr insisted that anyone over fifty who was a candidate for his valve must receive a coronary angiogram. This procedure was not being performed at the University of Oregon. To learn the technique, Judkins visited Mason Sones at the Cleveland Clinic, where coronary arteriography was being pioneered. Judkins brought the Sones technique to Oregon and used it on patients scheduled for valve implantation.

Soon Judkins grew to dislike the time-consuming Sones brachial artery cut-down approach for coronary angiography and developed his own technique, which required considerably less time. Still, the Sones contact showed Judkins that the open, tapered-tip catheter could be coaxed into the coronary ostia and that high-quality coronary angiograms could be obtained with only a small volume of contrast medium.

The Swedish Influence

At the age of forty-three, Judkins, with encouragement from Charles Dotter, accepted a fellowship to study selective angiography at the University of Lund, Sweden.

Melvin and his wife Eileen arrived in Sweden on Christmas Day, 1965. He began study under the tutelage of Olle Olsson and Erik Boijsen. In 1966, Judkins and Boijsen developed the hook-tail (U-shaped) catheter for the safe, rapid injection of contrast medium into the left ventricle. Judkins also came into contact with Olin's pioneering work on the flow-versus-pressure characteristics of catheters. He also learned the technique of placing a stiff wire on x-ray film, bending the wire to conform to the vessel, and then shaping a catheter over the wire.

While in Sweden, Judkins visited radiologists in Stockholm, Göteborg, and Uppsala. In Lund, he published three papers with Boijsen—one on the hook-tail catheter, one on angiography of hepatic rupture, and one on angiography of pheochromocytoma.

Research with Dotter

On his return to the University of Oregon in December 1966, Judkins started a four-year period of productive research in collaboration with Charles Dotter, chairman of the department of radiology. At this time, angiocardiography was transferred to the radiology department, and a new laboratory was created with Judkins as its director. Here, in the environment of encouragement, Judkins developed his small-radius J catheter for easy passage up tortuous vessels, his pigtail catheter for safe injection of contrast media into the ventricles, and his left and right coronary artery catheters.

In the construction of the two coronary artery catheters, Judkins was assisted by x-ray technologist Richard Stueve and engineer Robert Stevens of Cordis. Stueve fabricated catheters for Judkins; Stevens modified Judkins' catheters with stainless steel braid to provide even more torque control and strength for the new Judkins polyurethane catheters.

It is interesting to note that in a 1968 paper Judkins wrote, "The technique [percutaneous transfemoral selective coronary arteriography] can be rapidly mastered by those proficient in visceral angiography and with a little introspection and observation by those familiar with other coronary arteriography techniques." The connection here is obvious. The pioneers of visceral angiography were Boijsen and his colleagues at Lund, where Judkins had spent one year. The pioneer of the coronary arteriographic technique was Sones, whom Judkins had visited.

Judkins was at the peak of his productivity in 1968, publishing his personal record high of twenty-five papers during that year. By this time he had become professor of radiology at the University of Oregon.

Move to Loma Linda

In July of 1969, Judkins accepted the chairmanship of the Department of Radiological Sciences at his alma mater, Loma Linda University. This move was not unusual because Judkins was very fond of Loma Linda and wanted to do all he could for his church-supported university. The decision to leave Oregon was difficult, coming at the high point of his career when he had risen to the position of full professor and had built an outstanding angiographic laboratory.

For five months, Judkins made frequent trips from Oregon to Loma Linda, where he was busy reorganizing the radiology department, purchasing equipment, and recruiting and training staff. He moved to Loma Linda in January 1970, and the first coronary angiogram was performed early in November 1971.

Judkins threw himself into his work at Loma Linda just as he had during his practice years earlier in Antioch. He started work at 6:00 a.m. and held a conference on the angiograms to be done that day. In the evenings, he returned to the laboratory to preview the next day's cases and review previous cases. He always met with his patients the night before a procedure, explaining to them what he would do and outlining risks and benefits. After the procedure, he reviewed results with the patients. The pace was hectic—the interns called the coronary rotation "the slave service."

Awards and Recognition

Judkins received recognition for his contributions to coronary angiography from many prestigious groups. The Radiological Society of North America presented him with a Merit for Basic Research award in 1965. The Silver Medal for Distinguished Achievement was awarded to him in 1970 by the American Heart Association. The Clinical Investigator of the Year Award was bestowed on him in 1972 by the Walter E. Macpherson Society of Loma Linda University, which also named him Alumnus of the Year. He received the Distinguished Achievement Award from the American Heart Association in 1984. Numerous other awards were presented for his scientific exhibits.

Judkins was a member of seventeen professional societies and eleven national committees that dealt with various aspects of radiology. He was an officer in many national societies and served as president of two. He was a founding member of the Society for Cardiac Angiography, was its president in 1981, and was a life member of its board of trustees. He served as an editor for three journals and was a fellow of the American College of Cardiology, the American College of Radiology, and the Society for Cardiac Angiography.

Suffers Stroke

For eight years at Loma Linda, all went well. Then on January 12, 1978, Judkins suffered a stroke that left him handicapped. However, it did not remove him from the radiology scene. With his wife's assistance, he continued to publish a considerable number of papers and book chapters. He spent most of his time at home and enjoyed frequent contacts with colleagues, with whom he had had little time for visiting while at work. His impairment prevented him from participating in his many hobbies, which were drafting, flying, photography, carpentry, cabinet-making, electric wiring, and working with model trains. His hobby as an amateur radio operator was also denied him. Although able to do some gardening, he tired easily. Figure 6 is a photograph of Judkins in his later years at Loma Linda.

Judkins died in his sleep on January 28, 1985. In his eulogy, he was remembered as a clinical scientist and a dedicated teacher who was extremely unselfish in sharing his knowledge and skill with others. His greatest pride and satisfaction came from a job well done. Perhaps most important, he left the world of diagnostic angiography in a "better shape" than he found it.

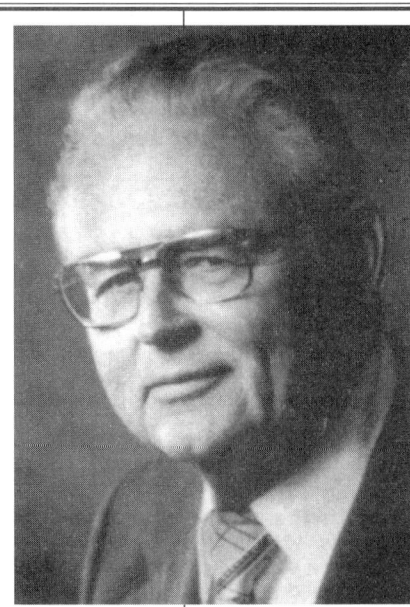

Fig. 6. Melvin P. Judkins, 1922-1985.

The whole of science is nothing more than a refinement of everyday thinking.

Albert Einstein

CHAPTER 6: Charles T. Dotter

Taking Catheters into Intervention

Give him a speedometer cable from a Volkswagen Beetle, and out pops a solution to control the rotational characteristics of a catheter. He created wire guides from sterilized guitar strings and piano wire. One never knew what to expect from the inquisitive and creative mind of Charles Dotter.

Today we call him the "father of intervention," thanks to his many innovations and his zeal. Dotter (Figure 1) was electric on the lecture platform, sociable with his friends, and an absolute terror to many of his peers and unprepared interns. When he was working with a patient, however, the only thing that mattered to Dotter was the human being on the table.

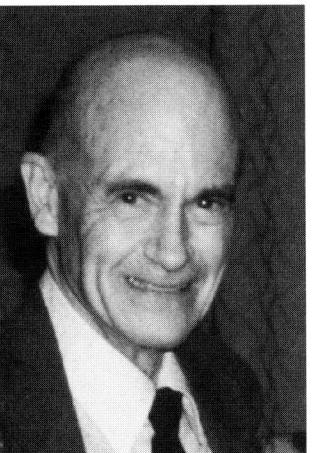

Fig. 1. Charles Dotter, 1920-1985.

Under Dotter's leadership, diagnostic angiography moved into interventional medicine. In the early years, it was necessary for angiographers to learn catheterization; in the Dotter years, the most important objective of catheterization became intervention. Yet he was a somewhat modest, unassuming man. When he talked about himself, he would simply say, "Dilation is my bag."

Crossing the Therapeutic Bridge

The story starts with a problem. It bothered Dotter that many conditions could be diagnosed by radiology but could not be treated. As was often the case, diagnosis was running ahead of therapy.

That changed, albeit slowly, after Dotter performed his first percutaneous transluminal angioplasty (PTA) on January 16, 1964. The patient was an eighty-three-year-old woman who had been bedridden for six months because of pain and infection in her left foot and toes due to peripheral vascular disease. A vascular surgeon advised amputation because of her poor cardiac condition. When the woman refused the operation, Dotter got his chance to prove the value of PTA. After the procedure, her pain disappeared, healing began, and she was able to walk on her own leg without difficulty until her death three years later. In a 1964 edition of *Circulation*, Dotter described the procedure as the transluminal treatment of arteriosclerotic obstruction. European radiologists, who enthusiastically embraced the technique, simply referred to the new approach as "dottering."

On March 9, 1964, at the University of Oregon Hospital, Dotter received a form from a surgeon requesting radiology consultation (Figure 2). The order was in reference to a patient whom the surgeon suspected to have blockage in the left leg. The surgeon, who wanted no radiologic interference, asked for a left femoral arteriogram and boldly wrote on the form, "Visualize but do not try to fix!!!" To some this might be viewed as a command; Dotter saw the challenge.

Arteriograms confirmed stenosis of the left femoral artery, but they also revealed stenosis in the right femoral artery. Dotter proceeded to dilate the vessel in the right leg. After all, he was not forbidden to fix *that* artery. He delighted in telling the story of how he got around the surgeon's order.

The Origin of PTA

Dotter's own words in the 1964 paper describe the origin of his PTA technique: "Despite the frequency and importance of arteriosclerotic obstruction, current methods of therapy leave much to be desired. Nonsurgical measures, however helpful they may be, provide the patient little more than an opportunity to live with his disease.

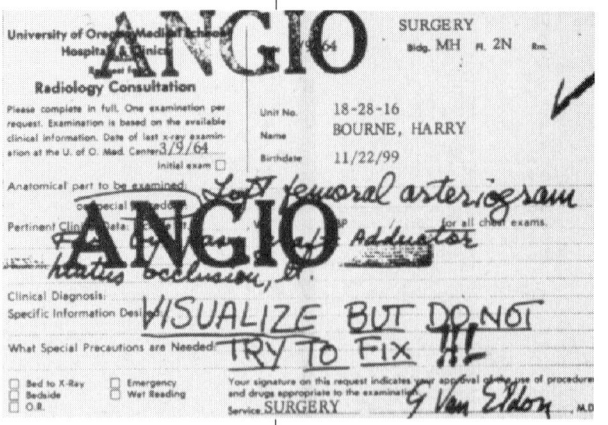

Fig. 2. This is the consultation request Dotter received in 1964.

"With these facts in mind, pursuit of a previously proposed approach has led to the development of a safe, simple, and effective technic for directly overcoming arteriosclerotic narrowing and occlusion in the arteries of the leg. Impressive salvages already achieved in otherwise doomed legs amply justify this preliminary report even though long-term follow-up observations are not yet possible."

In the Method section of his paper, he wrote:

The actual procedure is begun with downstream or antegrade femoral catheterization and control arteriography. A preliminary injection of 2,000 units of heparin is given into the artery, and under fluoroscopic control an ordinary coilspring catheter guide of about 0.05-inch O.D. is passed down the lumen beyond. A tapered, radiopaque, Teflon dilating catheter [radiopaque Teflon catheters were first produced by Cook Incorporated] of approximately 0.1-inch O.D. is then slipped over the guide and advanced until it too has traversed the block, thereby enlarging the pre-existing or newly opened lumen. The guide is passed across the atheromatous block without going through the wall more by the application of judgment than of force; both are often needed to effect the subsequent dilatation. Where desirable and possible, a second dilating catheter of nearly 0.2-inch O.D. is passed over the first.

Cook and Dotter

Bill Cook recalls his first encounter with Dotter: "In 1963 when Cook Incorporated was founded, we were fortunate enough to get space at the RSNA [Radiological Society of North America convention] at the Palmer House in Chicago. On Monday afternoon I was demonstrating to prospective customers how to pull tips on Teflon catheters when I noticed someone behind me sitting on a box. It was a short, muscular, bald man with darting eyes—I didn't know who he was, but he made me nervous. When there was a lull in business, I turned and asked if I could be of help, and he said 'no'—nothing more—and left.

"Just before we closed for the day, he returned and asked if he could use my blowtorch and 'borrow' some Teflon tubing. He said he wanted to practice making catheters in his hotel room. Thinking I had a real space cadet on my hands, I said, 'Sure, may I have your name?' He answered, 'Charles Dotter.'

"The next morning he was waiting for me with ten beautifully made Teflon catheters and my blowtorch. Remember, I had just started my business, and I admit that those ten catheters were sold to someone else for ten dollars each later that day. He was my first production employee.

"Every day during that week he returned. We discussed wire guide and catheter manufacture and what he thought the future would be for angiography. He became excited when he talked of his work, and yes, we discussed angioplasty. He hauled out the picture of his famous plumber's wrenches that we've all looked at so many times. Once started, his mind went nonstop.

"On closing day he appeared again at the booth and asked if I could come to Portland. I told him that I would. Before he left he said, 'You probably can't afford it, so I'll pay your expenses.'"

Bill Cook made the trip and discovered one of the finest laboratories in the United States. Cook continues, "When I arrived, I saw how his technicians made their own wire guides. Also, they were producing their own Teflon catheters using a recently purchased blowtorch and our Teflon tubing. Charles, by the way, was making the catheters.

"During this visit, he gave me a sketch of two telescopic catheters—10 and 14 French. I took the sketch home, ordered the tubing, and began producing the Dotter dilatation set."

Thus began a fruitful collaboration between Bill Cook and Charles Dotter. Dotter, however, availed himself of the resources of many manufacturers to develop new techniques for interventional radiology.

Before Its Time

Despite the success and acclaim Dotter enjoyed in Europe and elsewhere, "dottering" did not catch on in the United States until the mid-1970s. An additional decade would pass before Dotter received due recognition from peers in his native country. Many predicted that "dottering" was just a passing fad, and cardiovascular surgeons in general would not refer their patients to radiologists for these "radical" procedures, questioning whether treatment should be performed surgically by themselves or interventionally by radiologists.

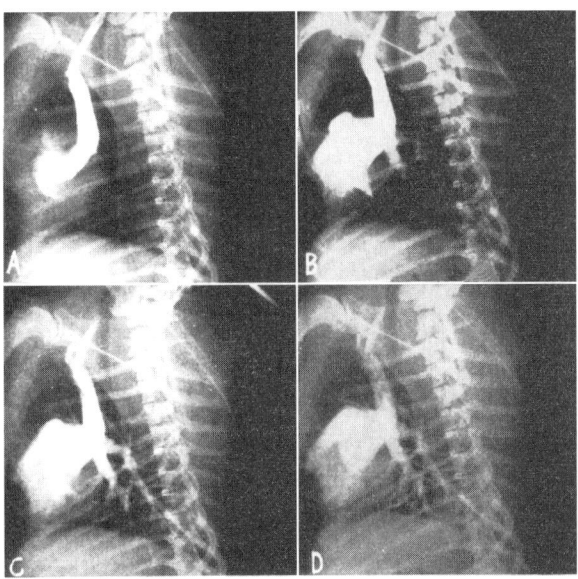

Fig. 3. Dotter obtained this angiographic study (left anterior oblique projection) of right-heart filling in a dog by using high-speed radiographic equipment. (A) 0.5 second after beginning of injection, (B) 1.0 second after injection, (C) 1.5 seconds after injection, and (D) 2.0 seconds after injection. All structures are normal.

Little-Known Techniques

In the words of Cook, "I existed in Bloomington, Indiana, from 1963 until about 1973 without a physician in our town understanding what Cook Incorporated did. That's how little was known about angiographic techniques and dilation and intervention procedures. Between 1963 to 1973, only about four hundred to five hundred people in the United States and maybe another five hundred in the world were doing these procedures routinely."

Many cardiologists and surgeons saw Dotter as being somewhat cavalier and perhaps a bit dangerous. However, they loved to hear him talk, and some would even wait for the opportunity to try to trip him up during his presentations. Nobody can recall ever hearing Dotter getting caught by his detractors.

As time went on, Dotter's so-called mad methods were proven correct. Andreas Gruentzig based his work on Dotter's methods. After Gruentzig shared his results with the medical community, Dotter's achievements in dilation began to be appreciated. Dotter's contributions resulted in near-elimination of exploratory surgery and brought about one of the great advances in medical history. There are many who feel that Dotter, Gruentzig, and Gianturco should have won the Nobel Prize in medicine for the work they did, which is now deemed "before its time."

Advances in Radiography

Dotter's vast knowledge of photography was a considerable asset in his creation of sharper angiograms. He knew that multiple rapid-sequence exposures were needed to follow motion accurately. He also knew that a very short exposure time was needed to freeze a moving object. With these considerations in mind, Dotter in 1949 secured the aid of the Fairchild Camera and Instrument Corporation to develop a rapid-sequence roll-film magazine capable of obtaining exposures at a rate faster than that obtainable with rapid-fire cassette-film changers.

The magazine held a 75-foot roll of x-ray film, 9-1/2-inches wide. Two high-speed intensifying screens and a parallel grid were incorporated. Lead shielding protected the film in the magazine from stray x-rays. The magazine weighed thirty pounds and exposures could be made every half second; each frame measured 9-3/16 x 9-7/16 inches. To illustrate the high quality attainable, Dotter presented right-heart angiograms at

0.5-second intervals, showing the dynamics of ventricular filling with contrast agent. Figure 3 is an example made with Dotter's high-speed radiographic equipment, which later became commercially available.

Focus on Exposure Time

Having solved the problem of rapidly acquiring x-ray images, from 1955 to 1956 Dotter focused his attention on the second most important aspect of high-quality radiography: exposure time. Blood moves with a velocity of 50 to 100 cm per second, and valve leaflets move even faster. Therefore, exposure times of a few milliseconds were needed to capture such quick motion. The shortest exposure time then available was 1/60 of a second (16.6 milliseconds).

Dotter developed an electronic switch with the assistance of Machlett Laboratories. The switch consisted of a negatively biased, power triode vacuum tube placed in series with the x-ray tube, as shown in Figure 4A. Exposure was made by delivering a positive pulse to the triode

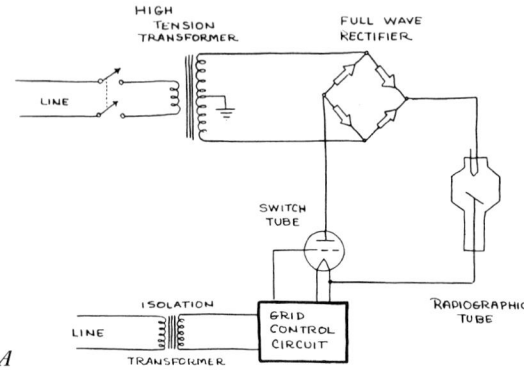

Fig. 4. (A) shows the circuit diagram for the high-tension switching triode Dotter used. (B) is an oscilloscopic photograph of a 3-millisecond x-ray tube pulse.

to make it conducting, thereby causing current to flow through the x-ray tube. Figure 4B presents an oscillogram of the current pulse that provided a 3-millisecond exposure time. At the 1956 Third World Congress of Cardiology, Dotter reported that he had perfected his system to provide 1- to 5-millisecond exposure times with x-ray tube settings of up to 100 mA and up to 100 kV.

Visualizing Blood Flow

In 1958, Dotter stated that it was possible to inject tiny radiopaque particles that would dissolve rapidly (within minutes) and could be used to visualize blood flow in combination with his high-speed radiography. He used the technique to study blood flow through dog valves but did not apply the method to patients. In a National Institutes of Health grant application, Dotter described the technique in colorful style:

> A long-range research project of the Radiology Department involves the development and use of injectable x-ray contrast substances, which take the form and role of discrete, tiny tracers within the bloodstream. As snowflakes trace the swirling patterns of the wind and smoke streamers plot currents in a wind tunnel, so these pinpoint tracers moving with blood can reveal the turbulence and eddy currents responsible for most heart murmurs. When we have learned enough to use this technic in our patients, we hope it will allow us to make x-ray movies of the sources of heart murmurs [which,

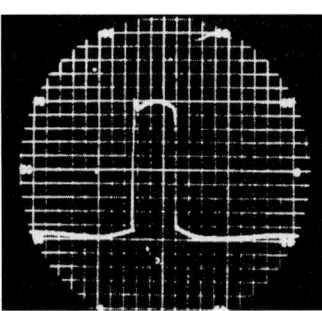

in themselves, are merely indirect signs of a damaged or improperly working heart]. Furthermore, x-ray pictures of minute spots moving through blood vessels also show promise of becoming the first relatively 'nondestructive' means for simultaneously recording the speed of blood flow at many different points in the body.

The same principle was used much later by biomedical engineers to study fluid flow around prosthetic heart valves in transparent mock circulatory systems. The visualization was provided by injecting bentonite powder; its movement was recorded photographically using polarized light.

Discovery of the Coaxial Catheter Method

To try out his idea for arterial dilation, Dotter proposed that a stenosed leg artery be opened in a cadaver. He obtained a long, stiff wire guide that was fairly large and not very flexible. (Dotter was making wire guides out of piano wire then.) One of his colleagues pushed the wire guide down the femoral artery past the obstruction, and it emerged at the ankle. Dotter placed a small catheter over the guide and passed it, then he placed a larger catheter over the first. Dotter soon tried it out on a patient.

At the June 1963 meeting of the Czechoslovak Radiological Congress in Karlovy, which was held prior to his first percutaneous transluminal angioplasty, Dotter referred to that cadaver experiment as follows: "Perhaps it is wishful thinking, but in any event I am convinced that the relief of atheromatous obstruction in small arteries can best be accomplished by catheter technics. A flexible guide introduced percutaneously into an artery proximal to an area of atheromatous narrowing can be manipulated so as to traverse the obstruction. A mechanical attack upon the lesion would then become feasible, perhaps by gradual direct dilatation."

Although there were deaf ears to Dotter's words in the United States, Europeans embraced the Dotter method. In 1967, Porstmann became the first in Europe to describe the use of "dottering," reporting 113 procedures in seventy-four patients. Other Europeans soon adopted "dottering" in their procedures. Thus the coaxial catheter method of widening a stenosis ultimately spread throughout the world.

Beyond the Limits of Surgery

In a 1964 paper written with Judkins, Dotter described application of the method to eleven extremities, resulting in marked improvement of distal circulation in six of the extremities and avoiding as many as four amputations. An addendum stated that since the paper had been accepted for publication, the number of patients treated had almost doubled and amputations had ceased. The authors concluded, "It seems reasonable to expect that the transluminal technic for recanalization will extend the scope of treatment beyond the limits of present-day surgery."

Not only did that happen, but in 1980 Dotter reported that "there are at least 200 scientific publications dealing with transluminal angioplasty, [and] more are forthcoming." He continued, "Not only peripheral arteries, but coronary, renal, visceral, and vertebral arteries, even the abdominal aorta, have been successfully dilated. Venous and arterial graft narrowings have been dilated successfully. Based upon published reports and equipment sales, it is estimated that over 15,000 such procedures have been undertaken!"

Evolution of Early Balloon Catheters

In 1951, Dotter turned his attention to the use of balloon-tipped catheters to study circulation. Note that this was long before Swan and Ganz introduced their balloon-tipped, flow-guided catheter in 1970. Dotter developed an ingenious balloon method that could produce a reversible increase in pulmonary resistance and completely obstruct a branch of the pulmonary artery. He mounted a rubber balloon (Figure 5A) near the tip of an 8.5-French radiopaque, double-lumen catheter. One lumen was used to inflate the balloon, while the other was open at the tip and could be used to measure pressure.

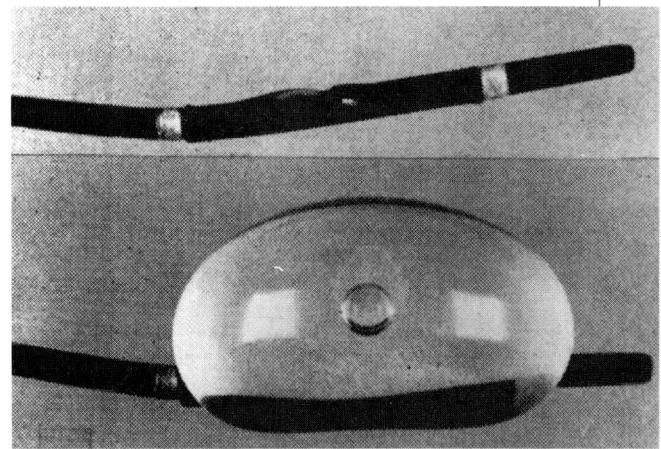

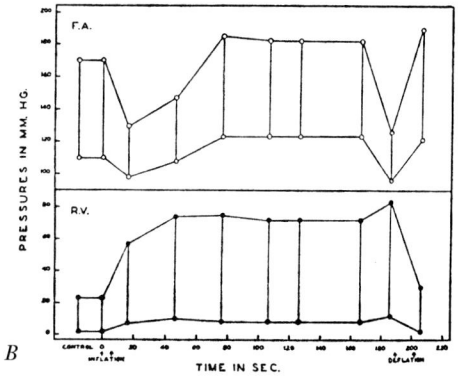

Fig. 5. (A) shows the catheter-borne inflatable balloon Dotter used to occlude the pulmonary artery. (B) shows femoral-artery and right-ventricular pressure before and after inflation of the balloon.

Dotter's objective was to create a method of testing that used the ability of the right ventricle to pump against a controllable resistance. In dog studies, he showed that he could triple the right ventricular systolic and diastolic pressures when the balloon was inflated. Figure 5B shows the femoral arterial and right ventricular pressure before and after inflation of the balloon in the pulmonary artery. He made no comment on the ease of placing the balloon in the pulmonary artery. Dotter appears to have been the first to place a balloon-tipped catheter into the vascular system.

Aortic Occlusion Method

From 1958 to 1959, Dotter (with Lou Frische) developed another use for his balloon-tipped catheter—selective coronary arteriography using a new aortic occlusion technique. Dotter pointed out that the rapid aortic-arch injection of substantial contrast media to produce clear coronary angiograms had met with variable success, so he proposed an alternative method. He knew the high blood flow at the root of the aorta quickly carried most of the contrast medium downstream, resulting in poor visualization.

Using fluoroscopic guidance, Dotter advanced his balloon-tipped catheter up the brachial artery until the tip of the catheter was one inch from the aortic valve, as shown in Figure 6. He then deposited acetylcholine into the aortic root through his catheter. A considerable amount entered coronary circulation and quickly reached the sinoatrial pacemaker, causing transient cardiac arrest. At that point, Dotter immediately injected Thorotrast contrast medium. With the balloon inflated, the only path for the contrast agent to travel was into the coronary circulation. Because all the contrast agent entered coronary circulation, splendid coronary arteriograms were obtained in seventy-eight dogs, all of which survived.

Although Dotter was enthusiastic about applying his aortic occlusion method to humans, he was cautious of the danger of ventricular fibrillation when acetylcholine is injected into patients on digitalis therapy. He cited a human fatality when acetylcholine was used to produce transient cardiac arrest. Most important, he said that if his aortic balloon technique was used, the operating team should be ready to perform an emergency thoracotomy in the event cardiac resuscitation was required. This particular study was conducted before closed-chest defibrillation and cardiopulmonary resuscitation were in widespread use.

In 1963, Straube and Dotter described an improved balloon-tipped catheter for coronary artery visualization by aortic occlusion. This device (Figure 7) used a single-lumen catheter for inflating the balloon and injecting contrast agent. The large single lumen provided a low resistance path for the viscous contrast medium. A unique arrangement of lateral holes in the catheter allowed the balloon to inflate before much contrast agent emerged from the catheter tip. Ingenious as this device was, it did not attract much attention, probably because it soon became possible to catheterize the coronary arteries selectively.

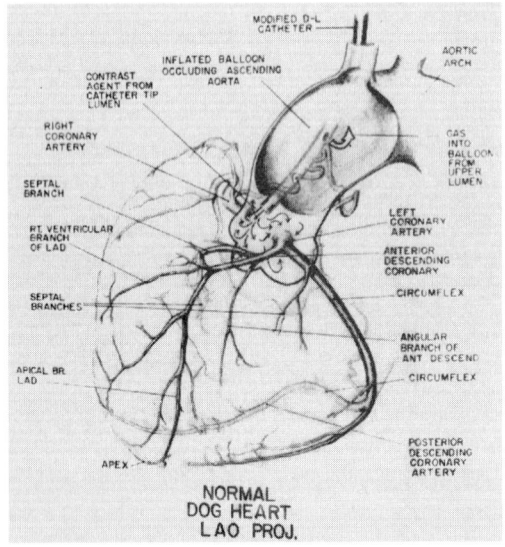

Fig. 6. Dotter obtained this selective coronary arteriogram in a normal dog by using occlusion arteriography. The left anterior oblique projection obtained at termination of injection of 5 cc of contrast agent was made during complete occlusion of the ascending aorta peripheral to the site of injection. The tracing was slightly augmented by referring to an additional but similar film of the same animal.

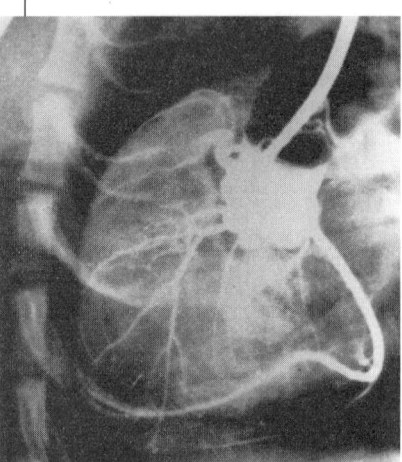

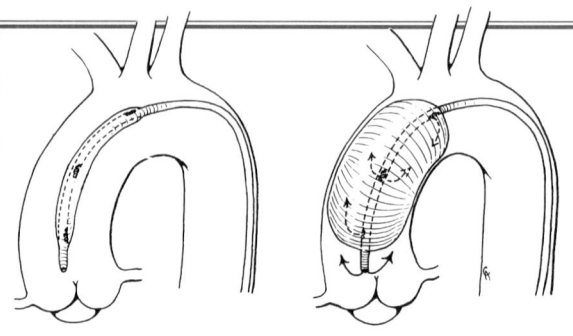

Fig. 7. These illustrations show how the Straube-Dotter single-lumen, balloon-tipped catheter works in coronary-artery visualization by occlusive aortography.

Flow-Guided Catheter

While Dotter was developing his balloon catheter, he also created a flow-guided catheter for the right heart and pulmonary artery. In 1962 he wrote, "During the time required to read this sentence, the reader's antecubital vein will be traversed by three or four billion red blood cells, virtually all of which will, within two or four seconds, reach the pulmonary artery. The free phase of pulmonary embolization is similarly brief. Why, then, does it require an average of ten to thirty minutes to pass a cardiac catheter into the pulmonary arteries? Explanation, if not justification, lies in the rigid catheter used for conventional venous catheterization."

After searching for a year for an ultra-flexible catheter material, he wrote, "Silastic, an inorganic silicone rubber, proved to be the ideal material for our flexible tubing. [Silastic X-30146, .08" O.D.] This tubing, percutaneously introduced into an adequate, unoccluded antecubital vein through a 12-gauge Robb-Steinberg angiocardiography needle, will, when advanced, pass with the aid of blood flow to and through the right heart chambers and into the pulmonary artery."

Figure 8 illustrates Dotter's catheter and a record of right-ventricular and pulmonary-arterial pressure made with this limp catheter. Anticipating occasional difficulties, Dotter stated, "The occasional tendency of the limp tubing to curl up rather than pass through the needle into the vein can be overcome through use of a nylon or wire guide stiffener inserted into the tubing prior to the procedure and withdrawn as the tubing is introduced. Impaction of the tubing should be suspected when there is difficulty in advancing tubing which has entered the vein but not reached the mediastinum. This can be confirmed by the ease with which saline can be injected. Repeated impaction indicates need for reinsertion into a more suitable vein."

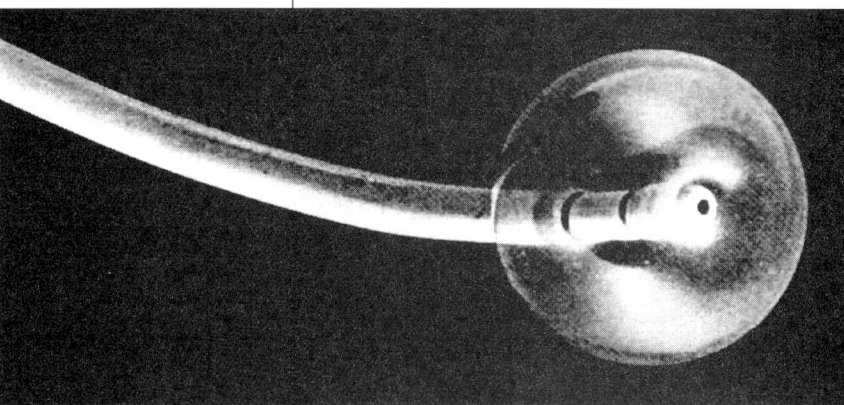

Fig. 9. Shows the Swan-Ganz balloon-tipped catheter with the balloon inflated.

The Swan-Ganz Catheter

Eight years later, in 1970, Swan and Ganz introduced a balloon-tipped, flow-guided catheter (Figure 9) that made the pulmonary artery as accessible as it had been with Dotter's limp catheter. Here, for the first time, was an easy, clinically applicable method of obtaining right-side pressures without the need of fluoroscopy to place the catheter. In addition, the technique could be applied percutaneously and was easy to learn.

The incorporation of a thermistor on the catheter by Ganz and associates in 1971 made it simple to apply the thermal-dilution method to determine right-heart (cardiac) output.

Dotter paid particular attention to the contributions of Swan and Ganz. He then proceeded to develop balloon catheters for other purposes.

Toward Better Balloons

Dotter was eager to make angiograms of smaller and smaller vessels. In 1972, he seized on the flow-guidance capability of the balloon-tipped catheter and coupled it with a curved catheter in an unusual way. He said that the method involved the injection of a long, radiopaque segment of silastic tubing through the lumen of a conventional preformed vascular catheter to extend the anatomical reach from so-called 'super-selective' targets [for example, the left gastric and gastroduodenal arteries] to what could be called ultraselective targets [smaller and more distant branches]."

Dotter had discovered that small-diameter, thin-walled, radiopaque silastic tubing could be easily advanced inside any curved catheter that was designed for selective arteriography. Figure 10A shows such a catheter. Prior to assembly, Dotter cut the silastic tubing to a length that would allow

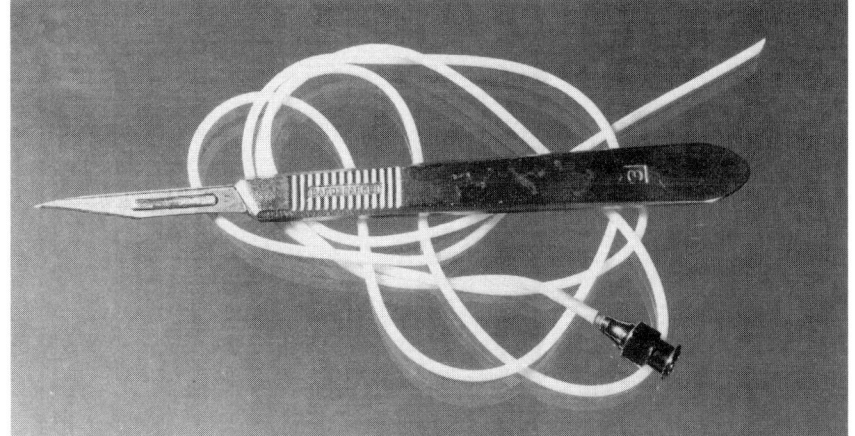

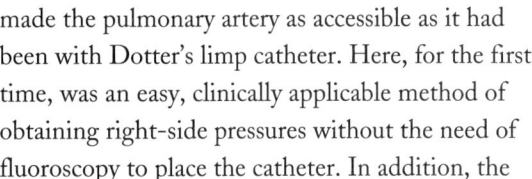

Fig. 8. This is Dotter's flexible catheter and a record of artery pressure taken with the catheter.

the desired protrusion (Figure 10B) and placed a locking collar on its proximal end. The preformed catheter was introduced in the conventional manner. When the tip of the preformed catheter was at the desired site, the contrast-filled silastic catheter (coiled inside the syringe as shown in Figure 10A) was ready for insertion.

When the syringe was activated, the silastic tubing was propelled through the curved catheter because there was no end hole in the silastic tube. When the tip protruded, it ballooned (Figure 10C) and the local blood flow carried the tip to the vessel of interest. Dotter did not clarify the location of the tiny hole that provided exit of the contrast agent. He enthusiastically wrote, "Not readily illustrated is the ease and rapidity with which the [silastic] tubing is propelled by the fluid shot from the syringe through the multiple curves of the delivery catheter." He said that he used this miniature "flow-guided" balloon to inject contrast medium into the splenic, hepatic, and gastric arteries in dogs.

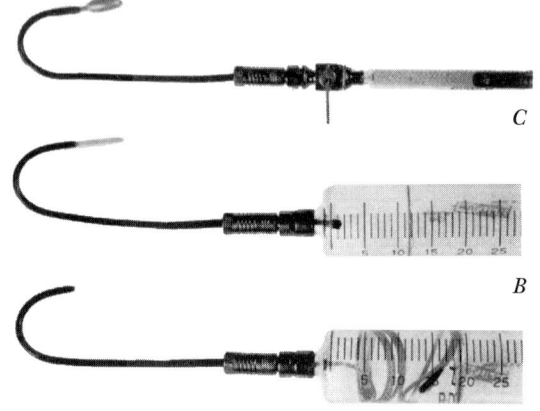

Fig. 10. Dotter developed this coaxial, ultra-selective balloon-tipped catheter to extend the anatomic reach of conventional curved selective catheters.

Fig. 11. Dotter's reinforced, balloon-dilating catheter (deflated and inflated) was never used in patients.

Despite Dotter's enthusiastic statement—"Catheter injection almost has to be seen to be believed"—and his comments about using the catheter for local deposition of therapeutic agents and vessel occlusion substances, others were not stimulated to use the "squirt catheter" (as Dotter called it). Perhaps, once again, he was ahead of his time.

Caged-Balloon Catheters

By 1974, Dotter was intimately familiar with the properties of balloon-tipped catheters and said, "Simple balloon catheters are not strong enough to achieve dilation of most iliac artery stenoses. An early design provided the needed authority by means of a woven fiberglass sheath that surrounded the balloon, but because of feared thrombogenicity [due to lack of smoothness], it was not used in patients." The balloon was illustrated in his 1966 paper. Figure 11 is a photograph of this woven sheath, balloon-dilating catheter.

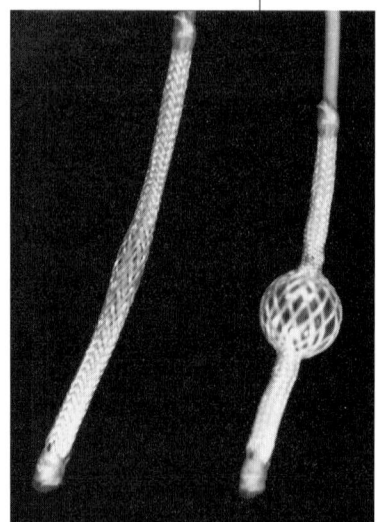

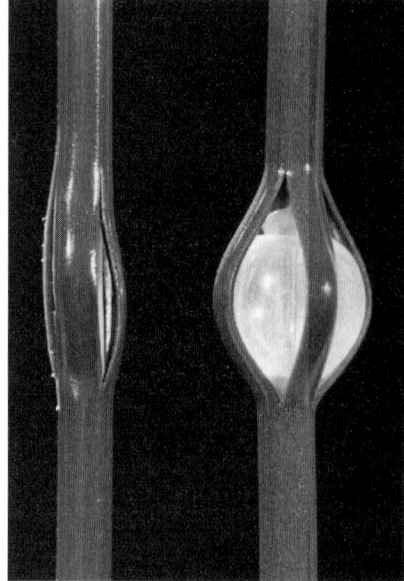

Meanwhile, in 1973, Porstmann developed a catheter similar in principle to Dotter's woven-sheath, balloon-dilating catheter. He called his device a "korsett balloon catheter"; it was made with material provided by William Cook Europe.

In 1974, Dotter improved upon Porstmann's corseted balloon catheter to create his own caged-balloon catheter (Figure 12). Like Porstmann's device, Dotter's catheter employed longitudinal slits placed over the balloon. When the balloon expanded, the slits opened and formed the protective cage. Dotter reported that the diameter of the caged-balloon segment could be increased from 3.0 to 9.3 mm when the balloon was inflated with 0.05 to 1.0 ml of dilute contrast medium under fluoroscopic view. The balloon was then deflated and moved longitudinally; the procedure was repeated as desired to effect a "stepwise dilation."

Writing in the *Journal of the American Medical Association* in 1974, Dotter observed, "By means of a reinforced balloon catheter, percutaneous transluminal dilatation was used to treat

Fig. 12. Dotter first used his reinforced (caged) balloon to dilate peripheral vessels. The balloon was reinforced by a thin catheter with longitudinal slits and inflated from a minimum diameter of 3 mm to a maximum diameter of 9.3 mm.

48 consecutive cases of atheromatous iliac artery narrowing. With no deaths and little increase in the time and risk of diagnostic arteriography, the procedure was successful in more than 90% of cases, giving immediate luminal enlargement and relief, as judged clinically, for up to six years, the maximum follow-up period."

Dotter wrote that this procedure required heparin anticoagulation and skill; speed was also desirable. He wrote, "Our caged-balloon catheter dilator system includes a thick-walled balloon mounted on a 60-cm long, 22-gauge metal cannula, terminated by a flexible, curved-tipped wire

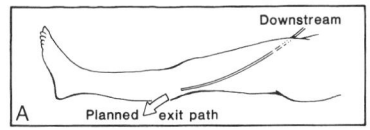
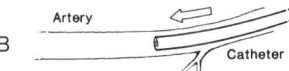
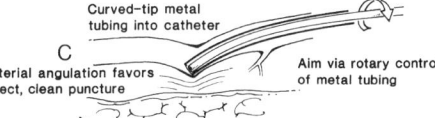
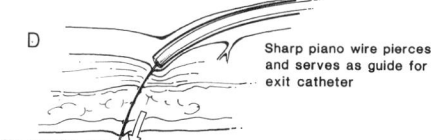
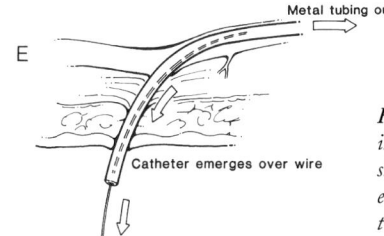

Fig. 13. These illustrations show Dotter's exit catheterization technique.

guide. Insertion of this balloon cannula all the way into a preslit No. 8-French outer catheter automatically positions the balloon within the cage 6 cm from the end of the catheter, beyond which the guide projects another 6 cm." Dotter said that with the caged balloon, a dilation equal to three times the catheter diameter was attainable.

It is clear that Dotter had conceived the caged-balloon catheter more than eight years before the 1974 publication date of his paper. He concluded in the paper: "On the basis of the results obtained in 48 treated lesions in cases followed up for the period of up to six years, percutaneous transluminal dilatation of localized atherosclerotic iliac artery narrowing by the technique described can be considered as offering the benefits of surgical reconstruction without the risk, pain and lengthy time of recovery."

Liver Biopsies, Exit Catheterization, and Coilspring Grafts

In 1965, Dotter described a liver-biopsy catheter in this way: "The instrument, similar in operating principle to a wire bottle opener, consisted of a 1.5-cm-long steel tube, about 2.5 mm in diameter, soldered to the end of a 50-cm-long coil spring of like diameter. The square-cut free end of the tubing was sharpened to a circular cutting edge. In use, a 45-cm length of large-bore polyethylene tubing was passed through an external jugular vein and the right atrium so that its tip could be advanced and placed in a hepatic vein, usually in the right lobe of the liver. The polyethylene tubing served as a guide and shield for the cutting spring catheter. When at the desired site, the latter was advanced about 1.5 or 2 cm ahead of the shorter polyethylene tubing, thereby passing through the vein wall and into the hepatic parenchyma. A corkscrew-tipped wire stylus was used for this [core extracting] purpose." Dotter used this instrument on dogs and, at the time, indicated that the instrument could be improved.

Exit Catheterization

"If something can be done by accident, it can be done on purpose." So wrote Dotter in 1969, referring to an inadvertent arterial perforation that occurred during catheterization. Based on this accident, he developed a technique for causing an intravascular catheter to exit the lumen of the vessel. This procedure, called "exit catheterization," is shown in Figure 13A.

Speaking of the technique, Dotter said, "The accurate control of the exit trajectory is 'built in' in the form of a long, blunt hypodermic needle slipped through, but not beyond the catheter [Figure 13B] to provide a relatively rigid intraluminal 'gun-barrel.' Unlike a rifle, however, this can be aimed by rotation, since there is a gentle, preformed terminal curve in the hypodermic needle. In addition, a desirable angular deformation of the artery is readily created [Figure 13C], thereby insuring clean mural penetration, rather than dissection. The actual penetration is accomplished with surprising ease by means of a long, sharp-tipped piano wire advanced through the hypodermic needle lumen, the arterial wall, and the surrounding soft tissue and the skin [Figure 13D]." The catheter was advanced as shown in Figure 13E.

Dotter applied exit catheterization to two patients. In the first, the procedure was used to

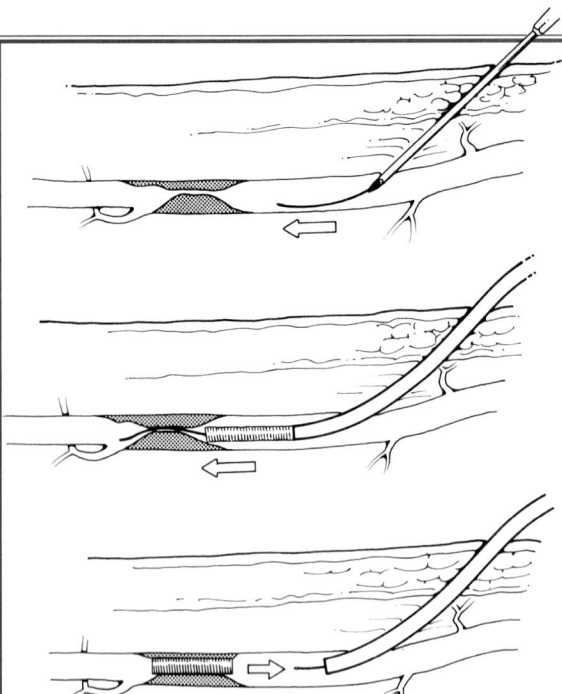

Fig. 14. Dotter's percutaneous method of implanting tubular vascular grafts.

Inserting Grafts

Some vessels that have been dilated often thrombose at the site and become narrowed or occluded. To remedy this problem, Dotter described the percutaneous insertion of grafts in 1969. His description of the technique (Figure 14) was succinct: "Using a suitable remote entry site and conventional techniques, a guide catheter is first placed so that its tip transverses the desired graft site. The tubular prosthetic graft and pusher catheter of similar cross-sections are then slipped on and advanced over the guide catheter until the graft has been seated as desired. Withdrawal of the former guide and pusher catheter completes the procedure."

In a twenty-five-dog study, Dotter evaluated the patency of plastic grafts, 1 to 10 mm long and 1 to 3 mm in diameter, inserted through the left carotid artery and placed in the popliteal or femoral arteries. He implanted polyethylene, polyamide, silastic, and Teflon grafts without anticoagulants and monitored their patency. In all cases, occlusion occurred in about one day.

Undaunted, Dotter then tried coilsprings of stainless steel wire wound on a mandrel. He constructed grafts ranging from 1 to 10 cm—some were left bare and some were coated with silicone—and implanted them into dogs. In describing the results, Dotter wrote, "Heparin was used until occlusion occurred, or for four days after grafting. A 10-cm, a 5-cm, and a 1-cm silicone-coated graft were found occluded the following day. Two out of three uncoated 1-cm coilsprings remained patent at two and a half years and two and a quarter years following insertion on serial follow-up angiograms."

facilitate the recovery of a Teflon-dilating catheter that had been allowed to slip beyond reach into the superficial femoral artery. In the second case, the method was used as an attempted alternative to arteriotomy in a patient whose completely occluded superficial femoral artery could be entered percutaneously only at a site below the origin of the occlusion.

In further commenting on exit catheterization, Dotter said, "The technique requires the professional skill and the high-quality radiologic equipment used for conventional catheterization, plus simple instruments, which can be homemade. The clinical role to be played by this technique remains to be conclusively established...it warrants the objective consideration of others."

Picking Up the Pieces

On occasion, guide wires broke, creating a very undesirable clinical situation. The pieces were difficult to remove and were sometimes left in place. In 1966, Dotter, Judkins, and Frische developed the safety wire guide in collaboration with Cook Incorporated. The result, Cook Safe-T-J guidespring (Figure 15), greatly reduced the incidence of breakage.

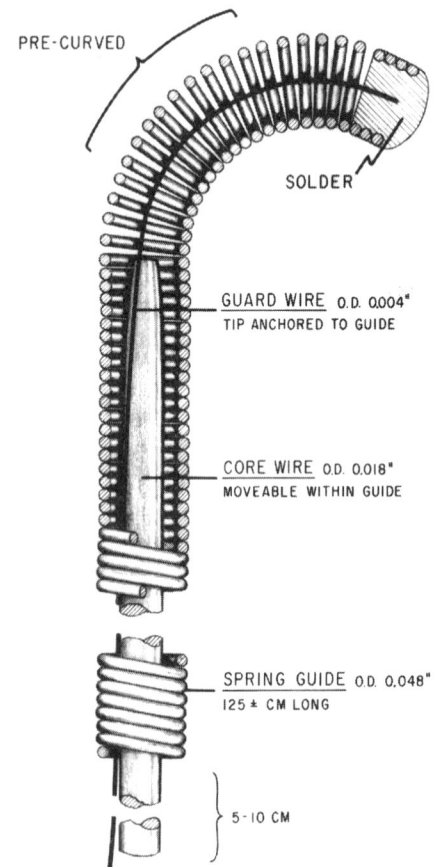

Fig. 15. Dotter and Cook Incorporated developed this safety guidespring with a guard wire soldered to the tip. It was designed so that in the event of breakage, the broken segment would still be affixed to the coilspring.

Dotter wanted more. In 1971 he wrote, "Based on collected case reports, the lives of at least 100 patients have now been imperiled by broken off bits of tubing or catheter guides lying within the lumen of the heart and great blood vessels. The complication is serious; of 62 cases of catheter embolization collected by Bernhardt et al, removal was not done in 28, and 17 of these died of related sepsis, perforation, thrombosis, arrhythmias, or myocardial necrosis. Removal of the foreign body is effective; no death was reported in any of the 34 cases where it was done."

The Loop Snare

Dotter devised a loop snare (Figure 16A) for retrieving broken wire guides and catheters and used it on twenty-nine patients. The technique of extraction consisted of first placing a guide catheter and inserting the snare into it. The size of the loop of the snare could be controlled by manipulating the ends of the wires (represented in Figure 16A by the letter "a"). Figure 16B illustrates a broken catheter segment that requires removal and is being captured by the snare. In Figure 16C, the loop snare has been tightened to bring the segment to the end of the snare catheter, ready for withdrawal.

In 1971, Bilbao and Dotter reported the first case of retrieval of an object from the gastrointestinal tract using the loop-snare catheter. The need arose when a thirty-six-year-old man had a nasogastric tube placed with its tip in the distal ileum. The patient tried to pull the tube out, and failing, cut it off at his nose. By peristalsis it soon advanced, becoming coiled and lodged at the ligament of Treitz (Figure 17A). Passage of an open-ended nasogastric tube with a loop snare to seize the wayward tube was ineffective.

Bilbao and Dotter cut a slit in the side of a retrieval catheter so that the loop snare could exit and be maneuvered to capture the end of the trapped nasogastric tube. When this was accomplished, they pulled the loop snare, wedging the target against the retrieval catheter. They then withdrew the catheter, bringing with it the 10-foot segment of nasogastric tube that the patient had cut off. Figure 17B illustrates the loop snare in the retrieval catheter, and Figure 17C illustrates the loop snare exiting the side slit and capturing the target (t).

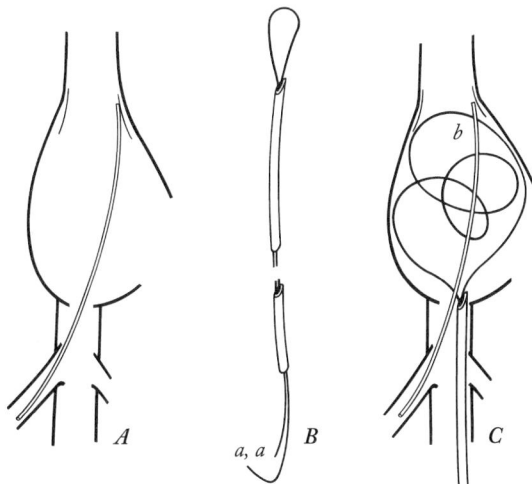

Fig. 16. The ends (a, a) of Dotter's loop-snare catheter (A) could be manipulated to create a single or multicoil snare. The loop of the snare (B) was used to capture a broken catheter segment (b). The loop snare was then drawn up (C) to bring the captured broken catheter to the snare and guide catheter for easy withdrawal.

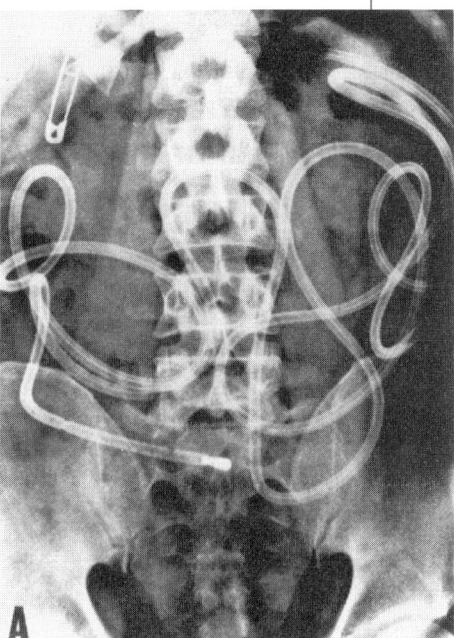

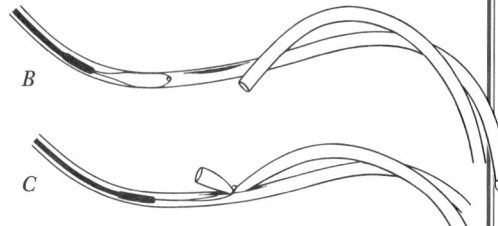

Fig. 17. (A) shows a swallowed, coiled nasogastric tube. (B) illustrates the retrieval nasogastric tube containing a loop snare that could be passed out through a slit in the side. The closed loop snare is advancing toward the target (t). (C) shows the target being captured by the loop snare.

New Devices, New Techniques

Having developed numerous techniques for selective angiography and controlled vessel occlusion, Dotter and his associates turned their attention in 1974 to clot lysis using selective catheterization. Conventional clot lysis used intravenous injection of about 100,000 units per hour of contrast agent and produced a hyperlytic condition. Undesired bleeding was a side effect. Dotter suggested that local deposition of streptokinase would concentrate the effect and require much less of the drug. In a study of seventeen patients with arterial thromboembolism, Dotter and his associates delivered streptokinase through a catheter at the clot site, after they first used angiography to locate the site. They found that clot lysis by selective catheterization required only 1/100 of the amount of streptokinase that intravenous use required.

In 1976, Dotter and associates reported intentional selective occlusion of blood vessels. Using a 6- to 7-French catheter to catheterize selectively visceral vessels in seven dogs, they then passed a 3-French catheter coaxially 2 cm beyond the large catheter tip for deposition of 0.5 ml of tantalum-opacified isobutyl-2 cyanoacrylate, which occluded the vessel immediately. They withdrew the small catheter and confirmed the occlusion by angiography with the larger catheter. They then applied the method to two patients, one with pelvic hemorrhage. The renal arteries were occluded in the second patient, who was on renal dialysis.

Expandable Arterial Stent

Dotter loved gadgets; he began toying with nitinol, which is an alloy with a memory. It can be shaped at an elevated temperature, cooled, and reformed. Reheating causes it to assume its original configuration. Dotter and his associates took advantage of this property to create an expandable arterial stent in 1983. A large nitinol coil was formed and, when cooled, reformed into a smaller coil (Figure 18A). When heated, it assumed its original larger diameter (Figure 18B).

The method of using the nitinol stent consisted of placing the unexpanded coil over a closed-ended catheter that had many side holes in the region of the coil. This catheter was placed inside another catheter for positioning at the lesion. With the coil at the lesion site, 20 to 30 ml of hot saline (140°C) was injected, instantly expanding the nitinol coil. The procedure was tested in dog femoral arteries. Dotter believed that there were many areas of application and suggested that the heat could be created in the coil by passing current through it. The coil could be easily heated by diathermy or microwave energy, neither of which would require electrical contact with the coil.

Just before his death in 1985, Dotter was conducting further studies on selective occlusion of vessels and retrieval of objects in the vascular and urinary system—using catheters, of course.

About Dotter

Dotter preferred to be called Charles, but many referred to him as Crazy Charlie. John Abele describes Dotter as a "classical, non-linear thinker who did much of his experimentation in his kitchen."

Charles Dotter was born in Boston in 1920. He attended grammar school and high school in Freeport, New York. He received his B.A. degree from Duke University in 1941 with a major in psychology. After obtaining his medical degree from Cornell University Medical School (New York City) in 1944, he entered military service, interning at the U.S. Naval Hospital at St. Albans, New York. He then took a one-year internship in medicine at New York Hospital, and he later became a resident in radiology there.

In 1948, he became an instructor of radiology at Cornell and in 1951 an assistant professor.

At the age of thirty-two, he accepted the position of professor and chairman of the Department of Radiology at the University of Oregon Medical School Hospitals and Clinics in Portland, a position he held until March of 1984, when he resigned because of ill health.

Introduced to Angiocardiology

Dotter was introduced to angiocardiology while at Cornell with his mentor, Israel Steinberg. In 1951, while an assistant professor, Dotter co-authored a 284-page book, *Angiocardiology*, with Steinberg. This book was published before image intensifiers were available and before Seldinger had introduced the percutaneous entry technique. *Angiocardiology* represented a monumental achievement. It covered equipment, techniques, advantages, hazards, indications, and contraindications for angiocardiography. In addition to numerous excellent illustrations, as well as Dotter's own sketches, the book covered history, anatomy, physiology, pathology, and therapy. Because the term angiocardiography was new at that time, Dotter and Steinberg defined it as "primarily a method for demonstration of gross anatomic change rather than functional abnormality. The latter may occasionally be inferred when secondary changes are revealed."

The authors stated with pride, "The usefulness of this book rests in large measure upon its illustrations. With a few exceptions, these have been prepared from material in our own files. No angiocardiogram reproduced in this book has been retouched."

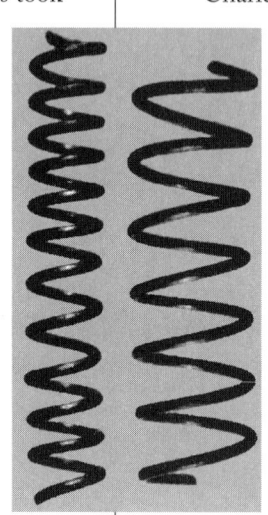

Fig. 18. Dotter's nitinol coil stent (A) could be expanded with heat (B).

A   B

A review of *Angiocardiology* prepared by Fell in *Surgery, Gynecology & Obstetrics* said, "This book is an extremely valuable contribution. The intrathoracic surgeon, cardiologist, and radiologist, particularly, will find it stimulating, educational, and of great help in the care of the patient in whom this procedure is indicated."

A review of the book by Sussman stated, "As a monograph on angiocardiography, this text will probably not be excelled for many years. It is obviously prepared by enthusiastic experts." Sussman did criticize the authors' use of illustrations from their own files and lamented the lack of perspective.

What a Plumber Can Do for Pipes

In Portland, Dotter's creative and imaginative mind was evident at every turn. His technical skill with instruments and his boundless energy were ready for the problems of the future. He brought an international perspective to the field by going to Europe to teach, to learn, and to share new techniques and knowledge.

He brought the Seldinger technique to the United States. He introduced many interventional practitioners to the U.S., including Josef Rösch

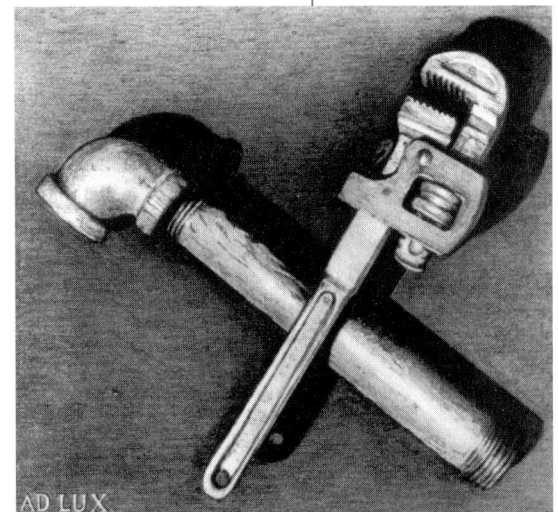

Fig. 19. Dotter sketched a pipe and wrench crossed like this to indicate that his activities resembled those of a plumber.

(Czechoslovakia), Werner Portsmann (East Germany), and Laszlo Horvath Hungary). He and others also worked to ensure the availability of tools for work in their own countries. International regulations made that difficult, but Dotter was not deterred. On a number of occasions, he smuggled wire guides to Rösch in the Eastern bloc. (Dotter hid them in the hubcaps of his car.) He also transported catheters across borders as pieces of tubing.

His personal view of solving technical problems is intriguing. In a 1981 edition of *Applied Radiology* Dotter said, "Between the idea and the actual instrument needed to implement the idea is a bigger jump than you might think." The fact that he was able to create early interventional tools out of everyday items—guitar strings, piano wire, and even a Volkswagen speedometer cable—is a tribute to his practical genius.

Dotter was maestro of the catheter, always seeking new ways to employ it. Yet he made his point humorously and effectively when he said, "My favorite conceptual trademark is a sketch that I did years ago of a crossed pipe and wrench [Figure 19]. It is a gross oversimplification, of course, but it means to me that if a plumber can do it for pipes, we can do it for blood vessels."

Papers... from Aneurysms to Mountaintops

Dotter was an excellent communicator, both as a lecturer and scientific writer. He made his points clearly and succinctly. He published 320 scientific papers; of those, he was the senior author on about half. The first paper on which his name appeared was published with Kuder in 1944 and dealt with vaginal delivery. The first paper on which he was senior author appeared in 1949 and dealt with congenital aneurysms of the pulmonary artery. That same year, he published eleven papers. During the next four years, he wrote about a dozen articles annually, with a maximum of fifteen in 1951. He continued that pace until 1982 when his publication rate was slowed—but not stopped—by ill health. Three papers were released after his death in 1985. Among his publications are twenty-nine book chapters and four papers that deal with teaching radiology to medical students.

Taking Medicine to New Heights

One of Dotter's papers (with Bilbao and others) describes a lightweight medical kit for mountain-climbing expeditions. Dotter and seven other climbers were going to tackle 18,008-foot Mt. Elias in Alaska. During the four-week expedition, they would not have radio communication, and the nearest aid was a thirty-mile hike and a plane ride away. The medical kit had to be complete and, since weight was a major consideration, as small as possible. The situation was ripe for innovation, and Dotter responded with creativity.

> **CLEAR COMMUNICATION**
> Bill Cook of Cook Incorporated, one of Dotter's close friends, was present while Dotter was performing an angiographic procedure on a man who was screaming on the table. Dotter yelled, "Shut up, you're screwing up my work!" The man suddenly got very quiet and barely uttered a sound during the rest of the procedure. Afterwards, Cook asked Dotter, "Do you do that to all patients?" He casually replied, "I do for the ones like this.... It's for his own good."

To avoid the need for bringing blood, each climber was blood-typed and cross-matched with the other seven climbers. Pragmatic as ever, Dotter wrote, "Thus we had on the hoof over 80 units of fresh whole blood from which emergency needs could be drawn, more than many blood banks boast."

Ever ready to pursue research whenever the opportunity arose, he inserted in his kit a "special, self-guiding heart catheter for the research measurement of pulmonary arterial pressure should anyone be so unfortunate as to provide the unique opportunity by developing acute high-altitude edema."

In the interest of efficiency, Dotter chose to include items with multiple uses; for example, "190-proof ethyl alcohol (4 oz.) for everything else, since it sterilizes skin and instruments, is useful in mountain sickness; one can burn it and, as a last resort, drink it!" Likewise, "cortisone antibiotic ointment relieves the inflammation not only of the eyes (including snow blindness) but also of the skin, outer ears, and lips."

The kit included sedatives and stimulants; cardiac, diuretic, and gastrointestinal drugs; antibiotics; laxatives; and tranquilizers. Also provided were minor surgical supplies, including scalpels, a hypodermic needle and syringe, ligatures, sutures, inflatable splints, dressings, and moleskin for blisters. Micropore tape was to be used for closure of minor wounds. Fortunately the expedition was without incident.

Pain and Peripheral Arteriography Study

Dotter was a thrilling lecturer; he knew how to make dramatic, memorable points. An excellent example is his 1982 presentation "Pain and Peripheral Arteriography Study," which compared patient responses to injections of both nonionic Iopamidol and hyperosmotic contrast media.

Herbert Abrams was there and wrote about it in a 1985 edition of the *American Journal of Roentgenology*:

> His paper consisted of a few sentences. At the beginning [he said], 'Let me turn this machine on.' At the end, 'That's all, folks.' In between, he played a tape recording of patients experiencing arteriography with the hyperosmotic agent. As the contrast material spread down the abdominal aorta into the iliofemoral system in these patients with aortoiliac disease, the groans, shrieks, and expressions of pain and dismay of all kinds reflected better than any arid set of quantitative data the full impact of the procedure on the patient.

The tape then continued with the recordings of another group of patients who had received the nonionic agent [Iopamidol]. For the most part, one mainly heard the physician, Charlie, inquiring solicitously, 'How does it feel? Does it hurt? Do you have a sense of burning?' And from the patients, not a shriek, groan, or even a single, 'Doctor, how long will it last?' The tape lasted a few minutes. Charlie turned the machine off, faced the audience, asked, 'Any questions?' And, when there were none, he sat down to a round of applause.

The authors are extremely grateful to Enid Ruble for supplying a copy of this remarkable audio tape, which Dotter frequently played to make his point to other interventionalists. One can easily hear the "clunk-clunk" of the film changer in the background. In addition to getting proof of patient contrast-medium preference, Dotter was timing how long it took contrast-media to get from the injection site (just above the bifurcation) down to the feet and was also looking for peripheral vascular disease.

Dotter asked the patients to rate the pain on a 1-to-10 scale, with 1 being no pain at all and 10 being the worst pain they had ever felt. One exchange went as follows during use of the high osmolality agent:

> Patient: "Let me tell you something . . . that ain't fun."
> Dotter: "On a scale of 1 to 10 . . ."
> Patient: "That's an 11-1/2."
> Nurse: "There's some discomfort down there, huh?"
> Patient: "Don't call it discomfort! It hurts like hell!"

Training Films with a Difference

While at the University of Oregon, Dotter produced an extensive series of training films, and one never knew quite what to expect. His films, unlike typical medical training films, were filled with humor and unexpected sights and sounds to capture and maintain the viewer's attention.

His film about transluminal angioplasty is a classic. The film opens with beautiful views of snowcapped Mt. Hood and the Willamette River as the soundtrack fills the room with the Mormon Tabernacle Choir singing "God Bless America." Having captured the audience's attention, Dotter proceeds to make point after point. "No reaming" is illustrated by showing a piece of metal being reamed, and "no drilling" by showing a drill going into a piece of metal. "No Roto-Rooting" is demonstrated by the animated image of a Roto-Rooter making its way through a sewer. When he says there is "nothing blasted," an atomic bomb explosion fills the screen; a dynamite explosion underscores "nothing blown out." For "nothing broken up," a jackhammer rattles noisily, and for "nothing plowed up," the famous Wile E. Coyote from the Road Runner cartoon series plows himself into the ground. The capper, "no stripping," involves a bit of female anatomy.

Wild and Wacky

Dotter was an avid outdoorsman. He scaled sixty-seven mountains, including all those over 14,000 feet in the contiguous United States. He even rappelled the treacherous Matterhorn unaided. Bill Cook spoke of Dotter's interest in the outdoors: "During the 1960s and 1970s, he would occasionally call and say, 'Let's go out west.'

"One time in Montana, Charles and several friends of mine from Indiana were having coffee at a restaurant in Beaverhead National Forest. All of a sudden Charles ran out the door with his camera. Some time later, we found him at the foot of a tree snapping pictures and talking to a young bear he had treed. Two other bears were watching off to the side. When we went back to the restaurant, we learned that the three bears were dangerous rogues that had recently been relocated from Yellowstone Park to the less visited Beaverhead Forest.

"Charles also took me mountain climbing—once. There we were on Three Fingered Jack in a blizzard—never again! He also tried to talk me into flying under a bridge so he could take pictures for one of his films. I wouldn't do it. Next, he asked if I would fly him near several mountain peaks in Southern Oregon. I did, but he couldn't take pictures because of the turbulence and snow. He was a bird watcher, artist, music lover, photographer, car buff, and mountain climber. He constantly challenged his body and his mind."

Cook remembers how Dotter arrived at a party in a tuxedo, fell in love with the owner's television set, which was broken, and proceeded to spend much of his time at the party taking it completely apart. The image of the TV repairman in a tux is memorable, whether or not he fixed the set. The point is that Dotter was passionate about everything he did.

Ross Jennings of Cook Incorporated remembers when Dotter was invited to speak at an international congress in Athens, Greece. He could not find out where he was supposed to stay, so he adapted. He called Jennings from the lobby of Jennings' hotel, came up to the room, and slept there for the duration of the congress. He never did find his own room.

Unusual Catheters from an Extraordinary Man

Dotter could not resist unusual catheters. Abele remembers an incident involving "a display [for Medi-Tech] that we used early on when dilatation

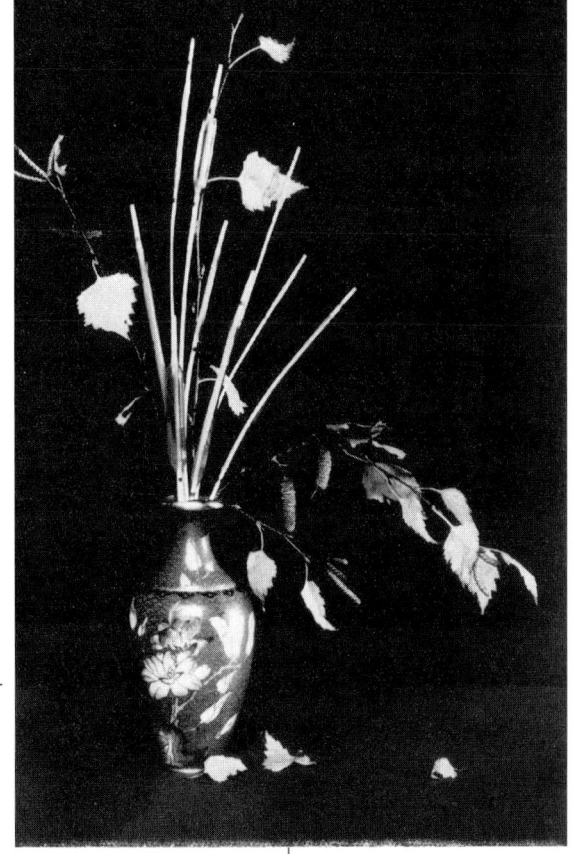

Fig. 20. *Dotter sent this picture of catheters arranged as flowers to John Abele as a joke.*

catheters were starting to become popular. We made a number of short catheters and put them in a vase and displayed them at our booth. The catheters disappeared at one of our meetings and we were somewhat suspicious that Charlie might have scoffed them up. A year later he sent me a beautiful framed picture [Figure 20] and the attached letter."

Dotter wrote the following to Abele: "This is a Christmas present and in a sense an expiation of a bad conscience. I found the depicted Medi-Tech sample catheters lying around on an abandoned registration table at a meeting in Las Vegas a year ago. Your detail man subsequently mentioned to me that he had lost them and I didn't own up to it. The least I can do is send you this [picture]."

Awards and Honors

Charles Dotter was an active participant in twenty-two professional societies and attained the rank of fellow in three: the American College of Angiology, the American College of Radiology, and the American Heart Association. He served on numerous National Institutes of Health panels, was chairman at many scientific meetings, and was a popular guest speaker at international conferences.

In 1963, Dotter received the Oregon Heart Association Scientific Award and the Silver Medal from the American Roentgen Ray Society. He received the Governor's Northwest Scientists' Award, plus citations at various scientific meetings. The Chicago Medical Society and the Chicago Radiological Society awarded him the E.H. Gribb Gold Medal. Gold medals also came from the Radiological Society of North America in 1981 and the American College of Cardiology in 1983. In 1984, the American Roentgen Ray Society recognized him again with a Certificate of Appreciation. Dotter was a Nobel Prize nominee in Medicine and Physiology in 1978. The impressive list of honors attests to the high esteem that his colleagues held for him.

Guttman Grant

In 1966, Dotter and Judkins received a gift of $500,000 from the Stella and Charles Guttman Foundation of New York. The circumstances surrounding the Guttman grant were reported in the November 1966 *Oregonian*. Stella Guttman had an obstructed artery in her leg and faced amputation because no New York physician was trained to perform angioplasty. Returning from a mountain-climbing expedition in Colorado with his son, Dotter received an urgent telephone call from fellow radiologist Philip Strax in New York. After hearing the problem, Dotter requested that Mrs. Guttman be brought to Oregon. The trip was not possible, so Dotter, his star pupil Melvin Judkins, and research assistant Harold Kidd went to New York to perform the dilation, which was successfully accomplished in forty-five minutes on June 28, 1965.

After the operation, Mrs. Guttman asked what the fee would be. Dotter and Judkins said there would be none, explaining that they were employees of the University of Oregon Medical School, the procedure was experimental, and they were glad to have been able to save her leg. Mr. Guttman said that perhaps he could make a contribution to their research and requested to meet with them. The medical team returned to Portland, and the Guttman award was made shortly thereafter.

In his final years, Dotter was anxious to develop a catheter for clot removal. John Abele describes Dotter's view of the device he was developing: "One product he viewed as his 'Holy Grail' was the expandable tip funnel catheter. He talked to Bill Cook and myself about it many, many times and we both tried very hard to come up with such a device. He was to present a paper at the Radiological Society of North America convention the year that he became confined to his bed. He was on the program, but we never heard his solution." Figure 21 is a copy of the program on which Dotter was scheduled. The funnel catheter was never developed.

Tuesday Afternoon • David Mayer Theater • Papers 361–366

Cardiovascular (Peripheral Vascular—Trauma)
Presiding: **Melvin E. Clouse, M.D.**, Boston, MA
Computer Code: K14 • 1½ hours • Give credit voucher to usher.

3:15 P.M.
361. **Percutaneous Embolectomy with a New "Funnel" Catheter**
    Charles T. Dotter, M.D., Portland, OR

The development of a catheter, the tip of which can be caused to assume the shape of a funnel within a blood vessel, places Fogarty embolectomy on a percutaneous basis. Its conduct, under visual control in the angiography laboratory, will reduce the risk hitherto associated with blind intramural passage of the Fogarty balloon catheter. Other applications of the funnel catheter, including percutaneous endarerectomy, are promising.

Fig. 21. This excerpt from the RSNA program lists Dotter's presentation. Due to ill health, Dotter could not present the paper.

In July of 1982, Dotter went to Milwaukee for his second coronary bypass operation, which lasted eleven hours. There was considerable scar tissue from his first operation, plus residue from radiation therapy administered to him for Hodgkin's disease in 1969, which affected his right coronary artery. His wife Pamela, a nurse, and daughter Jane cared for him at home during the last year of his life. He died on February 15, 1985, from pulmonary insufficiency.

Charles Dotter left behind a legacy of remarkable innovations and inventions. He helped thousands of patients. Just as great was his influence on countless other men and women throughout the world, who have gone on to provide comfort and life to a multitude of patients.

Teaching Technology

On March 15, 1990, one of the most important developments in the history of interventional medicine became reality—the Charles Dotter Institute of Interventional Therapy was established at Oregon Health Sciences University. The Institute is committed to life: both the lives of patients and the life of this great scientist.

The Institute provides advanced interdisciplinary medical education, research facilities, and patient care, focusing on the interventional treatment of disease.

The Dotter Institute is divided into three functional areas. The Clinical Section/Interventional Radiology is charged with continuing and expanding, in all disciplines, the angiographic and interventional treatment of patients. The Research Section at the Charles Dotter Memorial Research Laboratory for Interventional Radiology is responsible for research and development of interventional techniques and devices. The Education Section trains interventionalists and maintains a museum of angiographic and interventional history and cases.

Short-term fellowships of one to four weeks and long-term fellowships of two to three months are available to physicians from around the world, with tuition costs commensurate with length of fellowship. Fellowships allow the clinicians—radiologists as well as cardiologists, surgeons, vascular surgeons, urologists, gastroenterologists, pulmonologists, and gynecologists—to participate in interventional procedures.

Training of physicians, nurses, and technicians in interventional procedures is possible not only through personal instruction but also by transmissions through closed-circuit and satellite television. OHSU radiology residents receive the highest-quality instruction in vascular and interventional radiology. Referring physicians learn the advantages and disadvantages of interventional treatment so that they can provide informed alternatives to patients, resulting in increased public awareness of nonsurgical therapies.

The establishment of the Institute was made possible almost exclusively by private donations, including gifts from William A. Cook and Cook Group Incorporated. Major in-kind gifts of angiography equipment were presented by the medical systems divisions of Toshiba Corporation and General Electric Company.

There could be no finer tribute to Charles Dotter, the "Father of Intervention," than a living memorial that will perpetuate and expand upon his vision, creativity, dedication to interventional education, and commitment of service to humanity.

THE DOTTER-COOK PARTNERSHIP

Charles Dotter's inventiveness led to the development of many devices. Several of these were the direct result of his close work with Cook Incorporated, beginning with his first meeting with Bill Cook. Among the products generated through this collaboration were the following:
- Dotter Transluminal Dilatation Set
- Kerber Calibrated Leak Balloon Catheter
- Dotter Caged Balloon Catheter
- Curved Safe-T-J Wire Guide

In addition to the products Dotter himself devised, he influenced countless other scientists who continue to carry on his legacy at the Charles Dotter Institute of Interventional Therapy.

I have but one lamp
by which my feet are
guided; and that is
the lamp of experience.
I know of no way of
judging the future
but by the past.

Patrick Henry

CHAPTER 7: Andreas Gruentzig

Balloons from Switzerland

In his all-too-brief forty-six years, Andreas Gruentzig changed the face of vascular catheterization. He followed Dotter's lead, bridging the gap between diagnosis and therapy, using a radical new catheter.

Gruentzig (Figure 1) developed and refined percutaneous transluminal coronary angioplasty, an event so historic that King and Douglas listed it as one of the six important benchmarks in their book, *Coronary Arteriography and Angioplasty*.

Yet Gruentzig modestly announced his breakthrough in the following letter, published in the February 4, 1978, issue of *Lancet*.

Sir: In November 1977, we introduced a technique for percutaneous transluminal coronary angioplasty (PTCA). This technique consists of a catheter system introduced via the femoral artery under local anesthesia. A preshaped guiding catheter is positioned into the orifice of the coronary artery and through this catheter a dilation catheter is advanced into the branches of the artery. The dilation catheter [outer diameter 0.5–1.25 mm] has a sausage-shaped distensible segment [balloon] at the tip.

After traversing the stenotic lesion, the distensible segment is inflated with fluid [50% contrast medium, 50% water] to a maximum diameter of 3.0–3.8 mm by a pump-controlled pressure of 5 atmospheres [about 500 kPa]. This pressure compresses the arteriosclerotic material in a direction perpendicular to the wall of the vessel thereby dilating the lumen.

Gruentzig's letter continued with a brief description of his success with the procedure, verified angiographically, as it was applied to five patients. Word for word, the impact of Gruentzig's letter must rank among the highest of anything ever printed in medical publications.

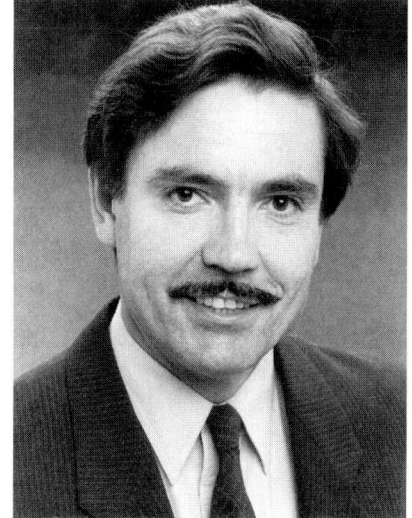

Fig. 1. Andreas Gruentzig, 1939-1985.

Coronary Angioplasty Comes of Age

Hurst documented circumstances surrounding Gruentzig's report in *Lancet* in Volume 57 of the *American Journal of Cardiology* (1986), as well as in "Benchmark 6" in King and Douglas' book (1985). The account, quoting Gruentzig, reads in part:

> Early in the afternoon [September 16, 1977] at a time when the anesthesiologist and the cardiac surgeon were available [to perform an emergency bypass if necessary] and no cardiac procedure was under way in the operating room, the patient came into our catheterization laboratory and was catheterized in the usual fashion using the Seldinger approach from the right groin and a Judkins-type guiding catheter. The chief of cardiology, the cardiac surgeon, anesthesiologist, cardiology and radiology fellows were in the recording booth to observe the procedure. The guiding catheter was placed in the left coronary orifice and the dilation catheter was inserted. Both catheters were connected to the pressure lines. The left femoral artery was also punctured and a sheath was placed. This was done to have arterial blood available to pump in via a roller pump through the main lumen of the dilation catheter into the coronary artery to perfuse the myocardium during balloon inflation. This had been shown to be effective for the prevention of acute ischemia during coronary experiments in dogs. We set the same system up for the patient because at the time we did not know how one would react to the sudden interruption of blood flow through the coronary artery when the balloon is inflated. I had planned to start the roller pump as soon as the patient would need it.
>
> After all these lines were installed and tested, the stage was set. The dilation catheter was advanced to the stenosis with no difficulty. The stenosis was severe but the catheter slipped through it without resistance. The catheter wedged the stenosis so that there was no antegrade flow and the distal coronary pressure was very low. To the surprise of all of us, no S-T elevation, ventricular fibrillation, or even extrasystole occurred and the patient had no chest pain. At this moment, I decided not to start the coronary perfusion with the roller pump.
>
> After the first balloon deflation, the distal coronary pressure rose nicely. Encouraged by this positive response, I inflated the balloon a second time to relieve the residual gradient. Again, the patient had no chest pain. After balloon deflation, the distal coronary blood pressure normalized as compared to the aortic pressure, indicating a good relief of stenosis according to our prior experience in peripheral arterial dilation. I pulled the dilation catheter back and tested the anatomic result with distal dye injection using the main lumen of the dilation catheter. My colleagues shouted from the booth that they also saw a narrowing in the proximal part of the diagonal artery and I should do dilation there as well. Seduced from their enthusiasm, I recrossed the stenosis again and went into the diagonal branch and repeated balloon inflation. Afterwards, I realized that there was no real stenosis in this artery and the balloon inflation was unnecessary. Fortunately, no complication occurred. I removed the catheters and the immediate control angiography in several oblique projections revealed a marked reduction of the LAD stenosis. There was no peripheral spasm or embolization. We therefore declared success.
>
> A few hours after the procedure, the patient phoned a newspaper, without my knowledge, and wanted to release his story. The reporter came to him but also asked me for further details and I begged him not to destroy me and the method by early advertisement of a procedure which had not proven to be effective at that point in time. I asked him to wait until more experience would have been accumulated.
>
> After a heated discussion in my office, we came to a 'gentlemen's agreement' to hold the story until more patients have been treated and until the first publication would have appeared in a medical journal. Fortunately, the press cooperated and kept the story secret until February 1978 when the first five cases were published in *Lancet*. Then the press took over and the story was given in all aspects and colors. By the way, the patient also had success otherwise, because he has now been symptom-free for five years.

By 1979, Gruentzig and his colleagues reported in the *New England Journal of Medicine*, "Over the last 18 months we have used this technic on 50 patients. The technic was successful in 32 patients, reducing the stenosis from a mean of 84 to 34 percent ($P<0.001$) and the coronary-pressure gradient from a mean of 58 to 19 mm Hg ($P<0.001$)."

The World Wants to Know How

Naturally, cardiologists, radiologists, and surgeons wanted details—more details than could possibly be found in scientific papers. To accommodate them, Gruentzig started to present courses in August of 1978 at University Hospital in Zurich. At the time, Gruentzig was one of the most sought-after personalities in cardiology, and many physicians from the United States went to Switzerland to observe the procedure.

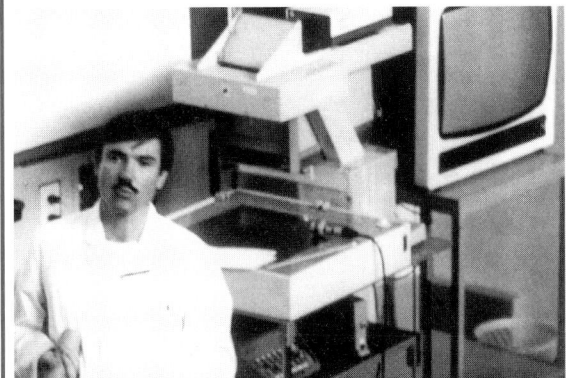

A

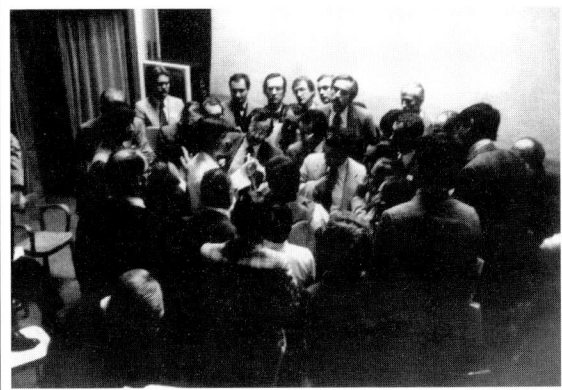

B

Fig. 2. (A) Gruentzig in his lab and (B) responding to questions from the audience at the University Hospital in Zurich.

Gruentzig taught four seminars in Zurich before moving to Emory University in Atlanta. He described the details of his procedure over closed-circuit television while performing balloon dilations on patients. Students watched the process on a large video monitor in an adjacent room. After each presentation, Gruentzig joined the observers and answered any questions on the procedure. Figure 2 shows Gruentzig responding to questions posed by the audience.

The Dotter Influence

Gruentzig's triumph came as a logical extension to dilation of peripheral vessels, accomplished in 1964 by Dotter and Judkins, in which coaxial catheters were used to effect the dilation. Balloons on catheters had been around for some time; they had their origins in urology. However, urologic balloons were not strong enough for vessel dilation. The idea exceeded the technology, but the challenge remained.

"Dottering" and Then Some

A number of researchers tried to develop useful balloon catheters. Gianturco dilated a femoral artery in 1971 with his first polyolefin balloon catheter. It was fabricated from a single piece of electrical shrink tubing. Unfortunately, Gianturco's first balloon-dilation patient died the night of the procedure when her wound opened as she slept; as a result, he abandoned the device.

In 1972, Porstmann invented an effective rubber balloon within a Teflon cage or "corset." Dotter and Judkins improved on Porstmann's "corseted" method, using telescoping and caged balloon catheters to dilate peripheral vessels. This procedure came to be known in Europe as "dottering."

Gruentzig, inspired by this technique, developed a catheter with a balloon near the tip. He started with peripheral balloons, which later evolved into coronary artery balloons. He also experimented with different materials to make the catheter thinner and more flexible. The original manufacturing technology for the polyvinyl chloride (PVC) balloons that Gruentzig used was developed in Denmark at William Cook Europe.

Credit to Dotter

Gruentzig, knowing about the caged balloon and "dottering," realized that everything he accomplished was based on Dotter's approaches and openly gave credit to him—something few cardiovascular physicians were willing to do until the late 1970s. In fact, worldwide medical

INTERNATIONAL AWARDS AND HONORS

Awards and honors came to Gruentzig while he was at Emory. The Radiological Society of North America accorded him the Award of Honor at its 1981 meeting in Chicago. In 1983, he received the Arthur Weber Prize in Mannheim, West Germany, and the International Recognition Award from the New York Heart Research Foundation. The Cleveland Clinic Foundation honored him with the Stouffer Medal, and the Texas Heart Institute bestowed on him the Ray C. Fish Award.

community acceptance of Dotter really did not come until Gruentzig gave his first publicized talk; then endorsement of intervention was nearly instantaneous. The importance of Gruentzig's blessing to interventional radiology cannot be underestimated.

In 1973, Gruentzig and his associates reported using Dotter's method to dilate stenosed arteries in the legs of twenty-five patients. He also catheterized renal arteries. However, he wanted to create a coronary artery balloon catheter that was small, strong, and did not need a corset.

With the advice of Hopff, a professor emeritus of organic chemistry at the Eidgenossischen Technischen Hochschule of Zurich, Gruentzig selected polyvinylchloride as a suitable balloon material. The balloon catheter was fabricated by Walter Schlumpf, husband of Maria Schlumpf, Gruentzig's operating room associate. Using this new dilating catheter, Gruentzig reported in 1974 that he successfully dilated peripheral arteries in fifteen patients.

Gruentzig's Dilating Balloon Catheter

Gruentzig discovered that when a soft elastic balloon at the tip of a catheter was placed centrally in a stenosed vessel and inflated, it expanded in the direction of least resistance and conformed to the shape of the stenosed region, rather than expanding radially to dilate the stenosis. It was clear that the hardness of the balloon after inflation was an important consideration.

Maria Schlumpf described Gruentzig's first experiments with balloon fabrication:

Andreas' idea to develop a catheter took shape in the beginning of 1972. His first idea was a balloon catheter, and one night we tinkered a model in his kitchen. Later we tinkered balloons made of different rubber materials, but the problem was always the same: under pressure the balloon made way for the stenosis and adapted to its form of a sand glass. It was a long but very exciting way to the useful balloon. We also experimented with other techniques and we also started at that time, for a short time, with the first laser experiments.

Dr. Hopff had no part in the construction of the balloon and catheter; but he was a very important man who had the right idea, [namely] which material [polyvinylchloride] would be useful for the balloon.

February 12, 1974, was the first dilation in a human being with a Gruentzig balloon [one lumen] catheter in a femoral-superficial artery and on March 5, 1974, the first in an iliac-communis artery.

Figure 3 illustrates the single-lumen catheter and one of the earliest patients who experienced dilation of a femoral artery stenosis with the new balloon.

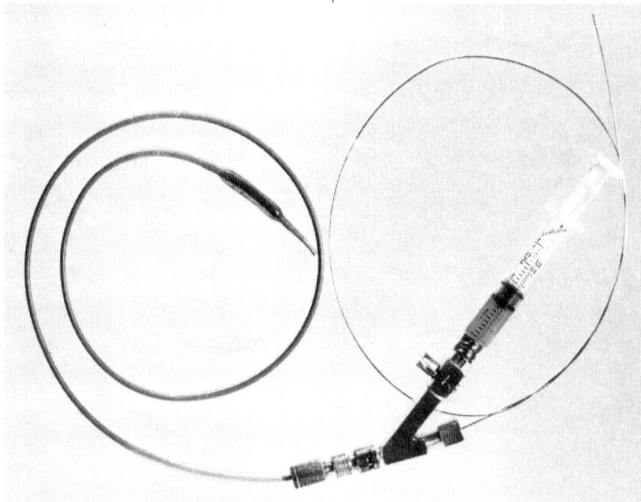

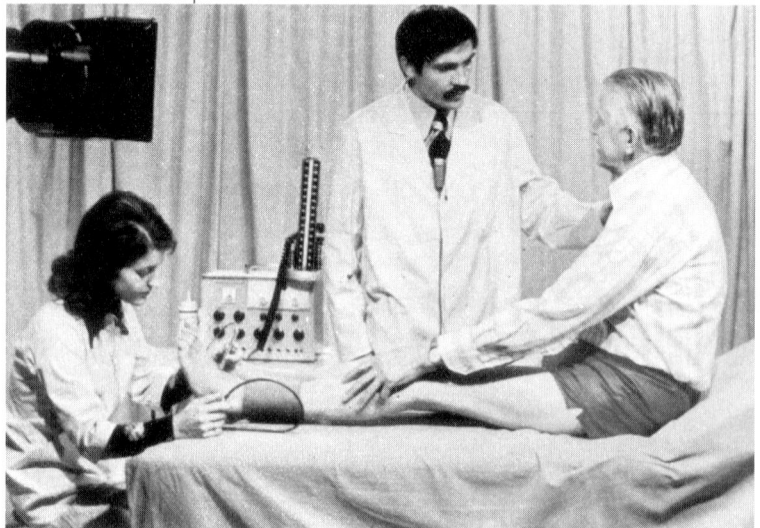

Fig. 3. (A) This is the single-lumen balloon catheter (1974) and a photograph of it being used to measure arterial pressure at the ankle of one of the earliest patients, following a femoral artery angioplasty performed with the Gruentzig balloon-tipped catheter. (B) Shown are Maria Schlumpf, Andreas Gruentzig, and the patient.

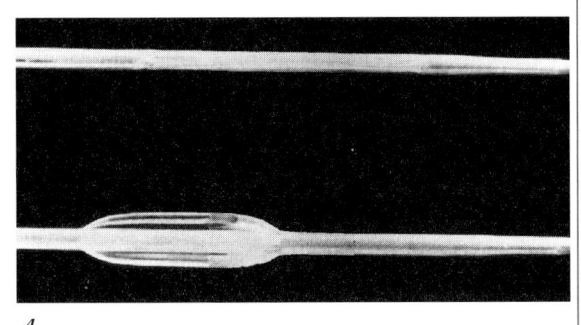

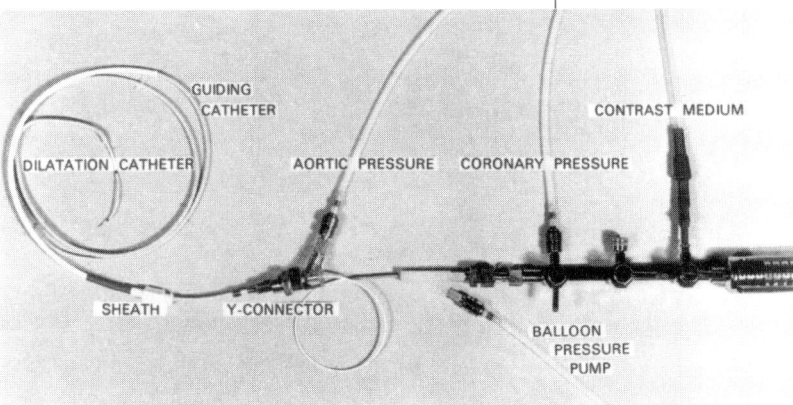

Fig. 4. *Gruentzig's balloon-dilation catheter (A) uninflated and inflated and (B) the original equipment used by Gruentzig in 1974.*

Seeing Double

After this initial success, in 1975 Gruentzig approached Christian Simonsgaard, the managing director of William Cook Europe, for help in the development of a double-lumen catheter. In January 1975, the first treatment with a double-lumen Gruentzig catheter was effected in an iliac-communis artery.

Schlumpf continued, "Until 1976, we made all the balloon catheters we used for the patients—also the early coronary balloon catheters we used for canine experiments—[making them] ourselves on the weekends or at night in Gruentzig's kitchen, together with Andreas' first wife Michaela and my husband Walter.

"In the middle of 1976 William Cook Europe and the Schneider Company took over the catheter production."

Figure 4 is an illustration of Gruentzig's 1976 balloon catheter for dilating coronary arteries, along with the accessory equipment. Figure 5 illustrates the Gruentzig catheter connected to a pressure injector to inflate the balloon with dilute contrast medium. Note the gauge on the left for monitoring the inflation process.

About Gruentzig

Gruentzig was born in Dresden, Germany, in 1939, when Germany was at war with its neighbors and World War II was soon to start. In 1945, just before the end of the war, his father was killed in Berlin. Gruentzig, his brother, and his mother were interned in East Germany; they later escaped to West Germany.

In 1957, Gruentzig received his B.A. from Thomas Gymnasium in Leipzig, Germany, and in 1958 another B.A. from Bunsen Gymnasium in Heidelberg. Afterward, he entered Heidelberg Medical School, where he presented his thesis and received a medical degree in 1964.

Gruentzig's postgraduate education reveals a broad spectrum of training, starting with a fellowship in physiology at Heidelberg, followed by a fellowship in epidemiology and medical statistics from the University of London in 1967. In 1969, he completed a fellowship in internal medicine from Max Rataschow Hospital in Darmstadt, West Germany, and moved to Zurich, Switzerland, as a fellow in internal medicine at University Hospital Polyclinic. From 1971 to 1973, he was enrolled in residency training there. In 1972, he received a fellowship in radiology and began active development of his balloon dilating catheter. In 1973, he reported using the catheter to dilate stenoses in peripheral arteries.

Gruentzig became a fellow in cardiology at University Hospital in 1973, and from 1974 through 1979 he was chief fellow. In 1977, he was appointed lecturer (docent). In September of that year, he performed his first coronary angioplasty; the research was supported by the Swiss National Science Foundation. During this time he also published his monograph describing the balloon for dilating stenosed peripheral arteries. The following year he co-edited a monograph with Zeitler (his teacher in Germany) and Schoop about peripheral artery dilation, including a short chapter on coronary angioplasty.

From 1979 to 1980, Gruentzig was physician-in-chief at University Hospital Polyclinic in Zurich. For his outstanding work in transluminal angioplasty, he received the Friedrich Goetz

THE GRUENTZIG-COOK PARTNERSHIP

The death of Andreas Gruentzig at the age of forty-six cut short a remarkable career that had already made a major impact on the field of radiology.

However, Gruentzig's all-too-brief association with Cook Incorporated resulted in one major development: the Polyvinylchloride Balloon Angioplasty Catheter.

At the time of his death, Gruentzig was working on a project that was carried on by other radiologists, in collaboration with Cook Incorporated, and ultimately produced the Gianturco-Roubin Flex-Stent Coronary Stent.

---

name first appeared on a scientific paper in 1962; the first paper that lists him as the senior author appeared in 1968 and was on epidemiology. His Award from the University of Zurich. The Third Symposium on Cardiovascular Disease awarded him the first prize at its 1978 meeting in Frankfurt, Germany.

Move to Emory
In 1980, Gruentzig accepted a position at Emory University in Atlanta and arrived in October, eager to establish the practice of percutaneous transluminal coronary angioplasty. At that time there were two cardiac diagnostic and interventional laboratories at Emory; when he died in 1985, there were six.

Gruentzig's publication record lists 232 scientific articles, of which he is senior author on more than one hundred. His first publication on cardiology appeared in the early 1970s. He published eighteen articles the year before he left Zurich, and about the same number each year after arriving at Emory. In 1984, he reached his peak, publishing thirty-eight scientific papers. Seven of his papers were published posthumously in 1986.

Not long after moving to Atlanta, Gruentzig met and married his second wife, Margaret. In 1984, he purchased an airplane to commute from Atlanta to his retreat house on Sea Island, Georgia. He had obtained a private pilot's license in Germany and later received a United States commercial certificate with instrument and multi-engine ratings. On October 27, 1985, the Gruentzigs encountered bad weather while returning to Atlanta from Sea Island. Their plane crashed near Forsyth, Georgia, killing both Gruentzig and his wife.

We are indebted to Gruentzig's immediate associates for personal information. Maria Schlumpf, who helped Gruentzig build and use the first vessel-dilating balloon catheter, said that Gruentzig was "a very great and special person." A collection of tributes from his colleagues at Emory was presented in the March 1986 issue of *Circulation* and the February 1986 issue of the *American Journal of Cardiology*. From these tributes, one can gain an intimate glimpse of his character. Hurst (who gave Gruentzig half of his office suite at Emory) viewed Gruentzig as "intelligent, creative, persistent, charming, charismatic, kind, thoughtful, confident but never arrogant, hard working, tireless, honest, filled with integrity, happy, secure as a person, and loving.... His cap was tilted to the side of his head as a signal to the world that he was accustomed to defying life's obstacles—he was ready for whatever might come."

Outpatient Angioplasty
According to Hurst, Gruentzig's next goal was to achieve outpatient coronary angioplasty. To demonstrate the procedure's feasibility, one day at 5:00 p.m. he had himself catheterized and then attended the departmental Christmas party. A second goal must have been laser angioplasty; according to Schlumpf, he had started preliminary studies while at Zurich. He was also preparing to work on stents when he died.

In December of 1985, the trustees at Emory recognized Gruentzig's contributions to medicine

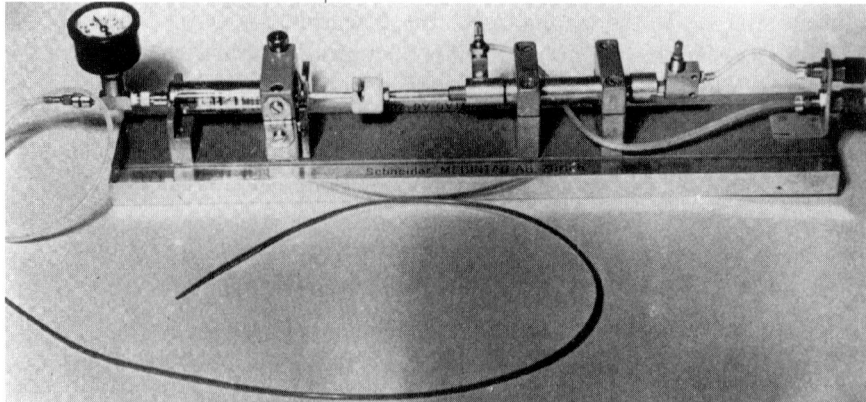

Fig. 5. Gruentzig's pressure injector was used to inflate the vessel-dilating balloon.

by creating the Andreas Gruentzig Cardiovascular Center of Emory University. John Stone wrote a moving tribute to Gruentzig in the October 16, 1988, issue of *The New York Times Magazine*. In it, the secretary to Spencer King, director of the Andreas Gruentzig Cardiovascular Center, related how on September 16, 1987, ten years to the day after receiving the first historic balloon angioplasty in Zurich, the original angina patient came to Emory for a follow-up look at his arteries. The secretary recalled, "Dr. King injected the dye...and on the big screen came this wonderful picture of arteries that looked—I hope mine look as good as his were—and the whole audience was just so stunned by this finding and everyone burst into applause."

Andreas Gruentzig made major contributions to balloon and coronary angioplasty. The development of his balloon dilation equipment made coronary artery dilation possible. One can only speculate about additional contributions Gruentzig might have made had he lived longer.

All interest in
disease and death is
only another expression
of interest in life.

Thomas Mann

Innovation in Devices and Procedures

Throughout his career, Kurt Amplatz (Figure 1) has continually conceived and created many new instruments and improved upon others. He is remarkably inventive, with an uncanny ability to demonstrate clearly the value of an innovative diagnostic or therapeutic device or procedure.

Although Amplatz's name usually appears last in the list of authors of a paper, there is no doubt that his influence is an essential ingredient in the research. His numerous appliances and gadgets are prominent in the catalogs of medical device manufacturers. His name is a prefix to many items, including a balloon-inflation device, balloon-dilator catheter set, stricture-dilation set, balloon-occlusion femoral arteriography catheter set, coronary catheter, dual guide introducer set, renal dilator set, ureteral stent set, biliary stent set, retention-catheter set, soft-shaft Malecot catheter, Malecot abscess-drainage set, anchor system, universal drainage set, vascular obstruction set, needle holder, and numerous wire guides.

Amplatz's name is also indelibly associated with the radiology department at the University of Minnesota, Minneapolis, where he has studied, practiced, created, and taught for more than thirty years.

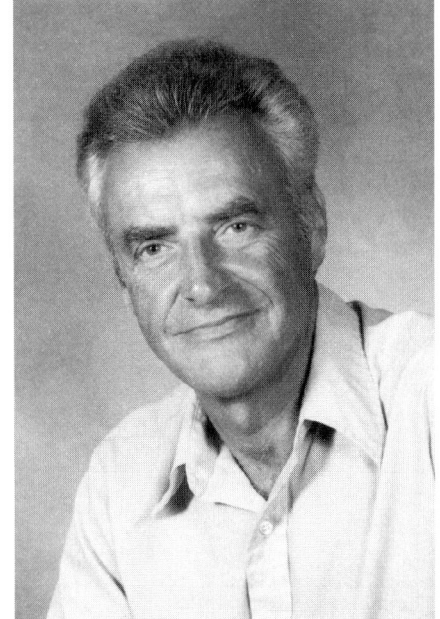

Fig. 1. Kurt Amplatz

Developing Better Images

Like many other angiographers, Amplatz studied ways to heighten the quality of angiograms and improve upon the tools of his trade. In 1960, for example, he said that the commercially available power injectors were expensive, cumbersome, and not suitable for *both* peripheral and coronary angiography. He set about to build an inexpensive, portable unit, shown in Figure 2A. The heart of this injector was a CO_2 capsule typically used to power soda-water dispensers. His equipment also consisted of a pressure regulator, which reduced the capsule's pressure to his recommended levels, and a stainless steel syringe. He illustrated the performance of his injector by comparing its pressure-time characteristics with those of the two commercially available and more costly units. The results are shown in Figure 2B.

Amplatz incorporated this pressure injector into 1963 research in which he attempted to reduce the problems of vibration and maintenance of uniform contact between x-ray film and intensifying screen. He placed x-ray film into evacuated, heat-sealed polyethylene bags and built film cassettes that could be changed at a rate of two per second. He also developed a syringe with a low-friction Teflon-gasketed piston to deliver contrast medium evenly. With this equipment and his CO_2-powered injector, he produced high-quality cerebral angiograms.

In 1977, Amplatz described more refinements to the CO_2-powered injector. His new model used disposable plastic syringes and produced a square-wave flow-velocity profile that assured uniform injection of contrast medium.

Crossing a Fine Line

Amplatz was also dissatisfied with the fine lines produced by the available eighty lines per inch intensifying grid. He solved this problem in 1967 by creating a circular, 12-inch diameter rotating Bucky diaphragm (Figure 3). Radiographs taken with the new device revealed no grid lines; however, close inspection showed faint lines near the center of the image. Amplatz eliminated these as well by placing two Bucky disks together, one on top of the other, with their grids at right angles.

Still feeling the need for high-speed, fine-detail film for angiography, Amplatz in 1968 developed an air-compression system for squeezing two intensifying screens against x-ray roll film, as illustrated in Figure 4A. Roll film passed between two intensifying screens that were mounted on stretched Mylar membranes affixed to air chambers 1 and 2. Gas pressure simultaneously applied to both chambers forced the intensifying screens against the film to make an exposure (Figure 4B). As soon as the exposure was completed, both chambers were evacuated instantly and the roll film was advanced, allowing for six to eight pictures per second.

Enlarging an Idea

For detailed visualization of the aorta-ileal-femoral vessels with contrast medium, Amplatz called attention to the value of 14" x 36" x-ray film. To solve the problem of storing film of this size, he devised a roll-film system capable of providing

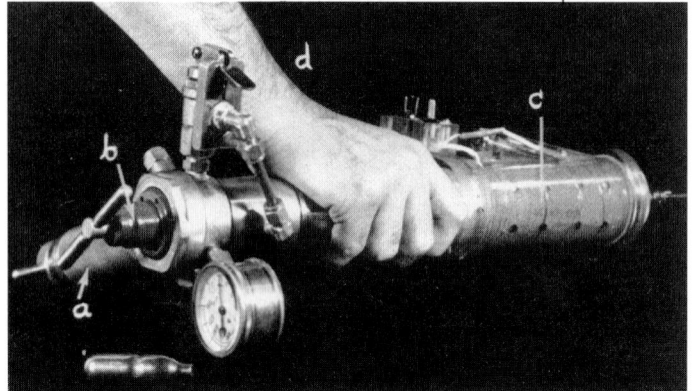

Fig. 2. (A) The Amplatz portable CO_2-powered injector for contrast media and (B) a graph of its pressure-time characteristics plotted along with those of two commercially available units.

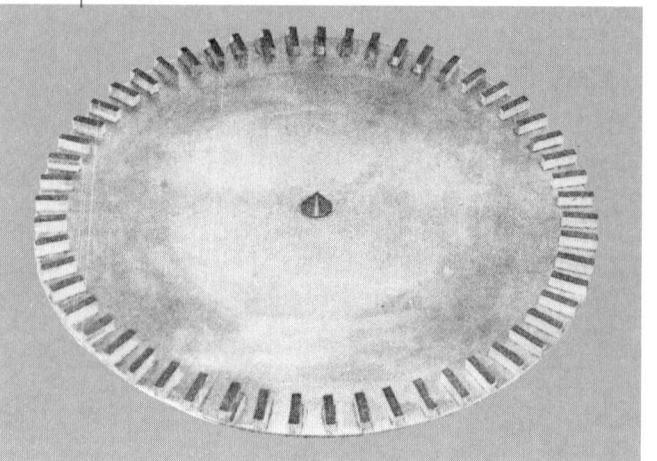

Fig. 3. The rotating Bucky diaphragm.

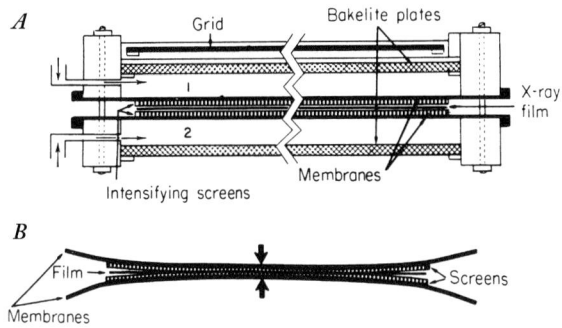

Fig. 4. This is the Amplatz method of providing a contact between two intensifying screens (A) that were mounted to stretched Mylar membranes (B).

14" x 36" images sequentially. His equipment (Figures 5A and 5B) used a 50-foot roll of 14-inch-wide film (A), loaded in a stainless steel transport magazine (B), and threaded over a highly polished roller (C) between the intensifying screens. The film was attached to a take-up spool (E), which rotated in a stainless steel receiving magazine (F), and was driven by a clutch-brake mechanism (G) and a motor (H). The space between the film and the intensifying screens was intermittently evacuated by a high-volume vacuum pump, a feature that provided intimate film-screen contact. At the end of the exposure, air was allowed to enter, and the downward motion of the compression plate (D) activated a microswitch, causing engagement of the clutch-brake mechanism for film transport. A program selector allowed the first exposure to be made after a predetermined amount of contrast medium had been injected. A footage counter indicated the amount of film remaining in the storage magazine. The exposed film in the receiver canister was cut off manually and taken to the darkroom for developing.

The film changer could be placed over an image intensifier, allowing fluoroscopic observation. The high-volume vacuum pump (I) produced a negative pressure of 5 psi, holding both screens in contact with the film. Intermittent evacuation of air and excellent screen-film contact was possible because a relatively long time was available for closure of the intensifying screen. Evacuation was accomplished by timing the x-ray exposure at the end of the timing cycle. After the compression plate had been closed at point B, the x-ray exposure was initiated by an adjustable time-delay relay for 130 milliseconds at the end of the compression cycle. With electronic timers, an exposure time of 0.10 seconds was easily available. From the time scale in Figure 5C, it would appear that radiographs could be made once per second, with a 130-millisecond exposure time.

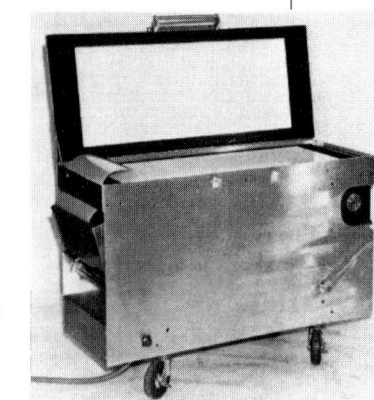

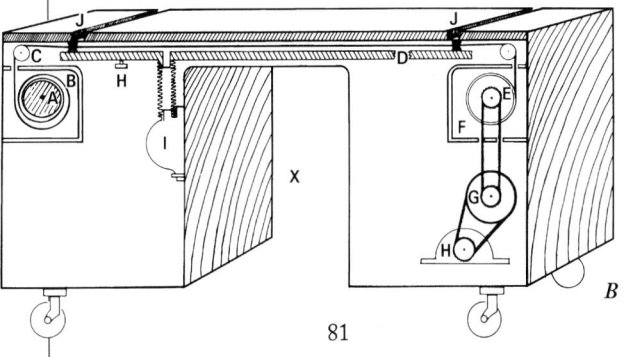

Fig. 5. Amplatz's 36-inch roll film changer with the cover open (A), ready for the threading of film (B). The time scale (C) illustrates the total transport time of 600 milliseconds, compression time of 400 milliseconds, and the x-ray triggered at the end of compression.

Fighting Thrombus Before Crisis

Thrombus formation was a potential complication associated with catheterization of the vascular system. Despite considerable efforts by many researchers to create catheter materials and surfaces to delay clot formation, the hazard of embolic complications persisted. Recognizing this fact, Amplatz decided to develop a thromboresistant surface in 1971. He pointed out that previous studies had reported the use of catheters with a heparin coating, but the coating stripped off easily during routine catheterization.

To solve this problem, Amplatz developed several different thromboresistant coatings made by combining heparin with different quaternary ammonium compounds. These coatings were smooth, waxy, and nontoxic and did not strip off easily during routine use. Toxicity tests were performed in mice,

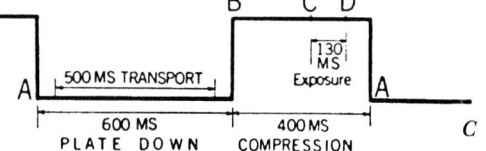

and clotting tests were carried out in dogs. Thrombus formation was delayed by about one hour in most dogs and by as much as three to four hours in some animals. Studies were also performed with small-diameter catheters in which the lumen was coated, with similar results. It was found that catheters coated with the Amplatz solution retained their thromboresistant property after seven months of storage.

In 1971, Frech and Amplatz developed a radiographic method of watching fibrin deposit on wire guides in the dog aorta. They applied the Amplatz benzalkonium-heparin coating to stainless steel wire guides and observed in animal studies that while five out of six untreated guides exhibited fibrin deposit in five minutes or less, the treated wire guides were free of fibrin deposits at four hours.

In a large patient study done in 1973, Cramer and Amplatz found that the thromboembolic complications associated with percutaneous catheterization were often due to stripping off the fibrin deposit during catheter withdrawal. Incidence of thromboembolic complication decreased when they coated the wire guide and catheter with the Amplatz benzalkonium-heparin.

To Clot or Not

Having developed a short-term thromboresistant surface, Amplatz in 1976 devised a simple and practical method to test the clot-inducing properties of catheter materials and surfaces. Catheters were advanced into dog aortas, left there for one hour, then withdrawn through a device that stripped off and collected the fibrin deposit. Figure 6 illustrates the Amplatz method of quantifying fibrin formation. Catheters were placed in femoral arteries and advanced into the abdominal aorta. A larger diameter catheter with a side hole and a filter at its end constituted the stripping and collecting device. After withdrawal, the filter was washed and the fibrin weighed. By far the most nonthrombogenic catheters were those that had been treated with a heparin coating.

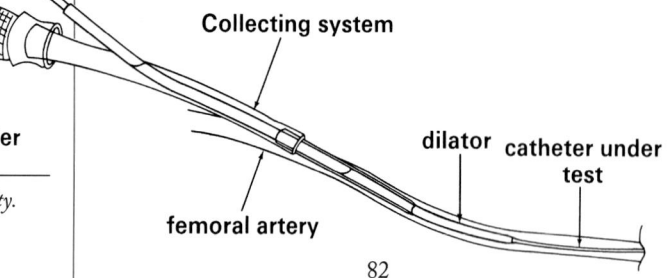

Fig. 6. Amplatz's catheter device for testing thrombogenicity.

Thrombus formation was of continuing interest to Amplatz. Realizing that thrombolytic drugs were expensive and slow to act, in 1989 Bildsoe and Amplatz developed a Roto-Rooter-like device for the mechanical dissolution of clots. The device (Figure 7A) consisted of an 8-French polyurethane catheter that ended in a metal capsule with two side holes. Inside the capsule was a tiny propeller, driven up to 100,000 rpm by a drive shaft that entered the catheter at the proximal end through one arm of a Y connector. The other arm of the Y could be used for fluid infusion or drainage.

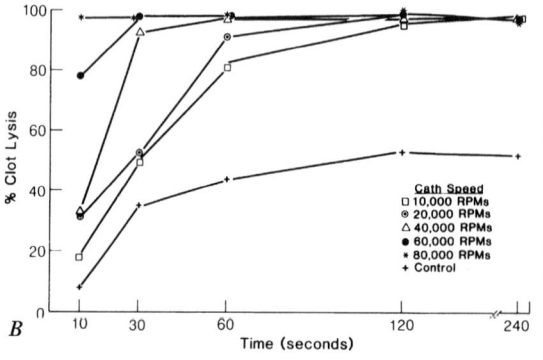

Fig. 7. Bildsoe, Amplatz, and others devised this mechanical clot-dissolution device (A), which consisted of a propeller rotating at high speed in the distal 1-cm segment of an 8-French catheter. The accompanying graph (B) shows the percentage of clot lysis versus time for different rotational speeds.

During in-vitro tests of the device, human blood was allowed to stand for twenty-four hours at 4°C to produce clots. The clots were removed, cut into segments 4-cm long, then weighed and centrifuged with saline in a test tube. With the propeller rotating, the catheter tip was advanced into and out of the clot. The catheter was removed and the clot residue was filtered, examined, and measured. Figure 7B shows that with high rotational speed, 100% of the clot was destroyed in less than thirty seconds. The largest clot fragments were found to be about 200 microns. Bildsoe and Amplatz likened the clot dissolution device to a food blender, repeatedly cutting particles into smaller and smaller pieces. They suggested that clot particle size could be reduced further and that the potential clinical application would be to destroy clots in bypass grafts. At this time, animal studies are under way.

Work with Therapeutic Embolization

Therapeutic embolization is used to control bleeding, to arrest blood flow to malignant tumors, and to close arteriovenous malformations. The interventional radiologist is uniquely qualified to exploit this technique, which can be performed percutaneously, and Amplatz actively researched ways to achieve therapeutic embolization in patients.

Working with Tadavarthy and others in 1974, Zollikofer and associates in 1980, and Herrera et al in 1982, Amplatz devised two techniques for delivering Ivalon (a polyvinyl ether foam) to arrest blood flow. The first utilized a compressed plug, which when delivered at the desired site, swelled and produced a clot. The second method used a suspension of Ivalon particles, the size of which was selected according to the vessel diameter to be occluded. (Ivalon had the advantage over Gelfoam by providing permanent vascular occlusions.)

Guiding Wires

A wire guide, which consists of an inner wire mandrel surrounded by a coil, must have two conflicting characteristics: It must be stiff enough so that a catheter can follow it, and it must be flexible enough to negotiate bends.

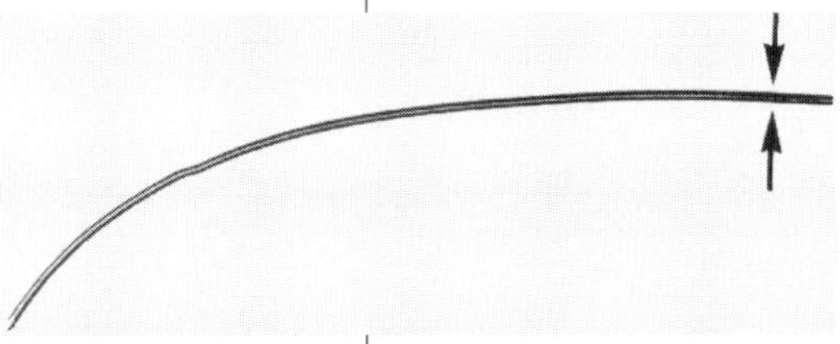

Fig. 8. One of the early stiffened guide wires with a floppy tip that Amplatz developed. It was stiffened by soldering the coil to the safety core at the arrows.

In 1985, when placement of balloon-dilation catheters, stents, and other new devices required the redesign of wire guides, Cardella and Amplatz created a stiffer guide with a mandrel that was soldered near the floppy tip (Figure 8).

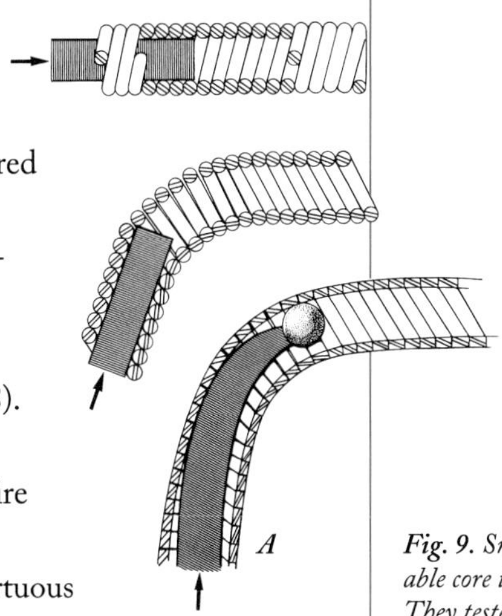

In 1986, Smith and Amplatz developed a flat-wire wound guide with a tapered moveable core, for use in tortuous vessels. The core was coated with Teflon and had a distal silver ball, as shown in Figure 9A. During maneuverability tests in curved glass tubes (Figure 9B), the Smith and Amplatz movable core wire guide negotiated the sharp bends better than the commercially available guides tested.

An extra-stiff exchange wire guide was developed in 1987 by Butto and Amplatz. Stiffening was achieved by compressing and soldering the coils of the wire guide to the core wire every 75 cm, as shown in Figure 10. To illustrate the efficacy of the new heavy-duty guide, Butto and Amplatz used it in studies of pulmonary valve balloon angioplasty in dogs and in studies of ductus arteriosus dilation in lambs.

Because standard wire guides could not be rotated readily, Robinson and Amplatz developed a torque wire in 1987. In a series of tests, they found that this wire guide passed through a multi-curved model in less time than was required for a conventional wire guide.

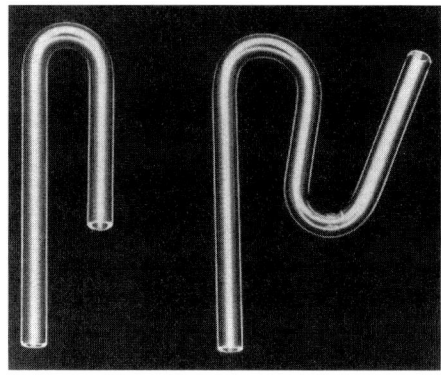

Fig. 9. Smith and Amplatz developed a guide wire with a movable core that was tipped by a silver ball (A) for tortuous vessels. They tested its maneuverability in glass tubes (B).

Evolution of Percutaneous Nephrostomy

After Seldinger described his percutaneous entry technique in 1953, the technique was used by many to explore the vascular system and pave the way for cardiovascular intervention. The ease with which a catheter followed the wire guide in vascular procedures spurred others to investigate the use of the Seldinger technique for nonvascular applications.

Beginning in 1954, for example, Wickbom pointed out that when blood flow to the

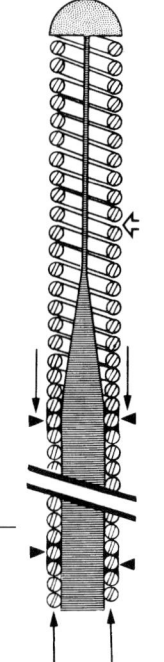

Fig. 10. Butto and Amplatz made stiffened guide wires by soldering the coils to the core every 75 cm. They stretched the distal 5 cm of the tip to provide flexibility and tapered the core wire to increase tip flexibility.

DOCUMENTING ENDOUROLOGY

Amplatz edited and contributed to the *Atlas of Endourology*, published in 1986. This book describes the instruments and procedures used in the field that he pioneered. The subject is explained step by step, with contributions from urologists to radiologists. Readers follow large, clear radiographs, explanatory sketches, and full-color anatomical plates. Amplatz wrote, "Gadgetry is an integral part of endourology," a circumstance borne out by the variety of catheters and stents illustrated. According to medical lore, the new instruments led to the comment that this marked the "end o' urology." Although that remark was certainly not true, Amplatz's contributions have helped to change forever the practice of urology.

kidneys was impaired and ureteral flow restricted, an intravenous approach to pyelography would be inadequate. To make the drainage system opaque, he injected contrast medium directly into the renal pelvis through a long needle. The next year, Goodwin and associates used a "catheter through the needle" technique for drainage. A decade later (in 1965), Bartley demonstrated the successful use of a wire-guided catheter technique for drainage, and in 1976, Fernström and Johansson reported dilation of the nephrostomy tract (employing an indwelling flexible cannula) for stone removal.

In 1978, Stables and associates reviewed the techniques used and the results of 516 percutaneous nephrostomies that appeared in medical literature, as well as those in a series of fifty-three of their own patients. They concluded that the method "is one of the most rewarding therapeutic procedures that the diagnostic radiologist has to offer...the vast majority of candidates for this procedure, some desperately ill and unfit for any surgical diversion, can be managed successfully without incident."

The Birth of Endourology

Smith wrote in 1979, "At least ten applications of percutaneous nephrostomy have been described recently at medical meetings and will soon be reported in the literature. . . . Because percutaneous nephrostomy and its various applications represent closed, controlled, diagnostic and therapeutic manipulations within the urinary tract using sophisticated urologic instruments, we suggest that the term 'endourology' be applied to such procedures within the urinary tract." Thus was born a name for the science: "endourology." At that time, Smith had just begun work at the University of Minnesota, where the environment was conducive to the development of new techniques and instruments now that percutaneous access to the upper urinary tract was possible.

Percutaneous entry into the upper urinary collecting system is achieved as shown in Figure 11. First the needle is passed (Figure 11A), then the wire guide is advanced through the needle (Figure 11B). The needle is withdrawn and the catheter is passed (Figure 11C). This principle is employed for drainage catheter placement, injection of contrast media, removal of stones, and insertion of ureteral stents.

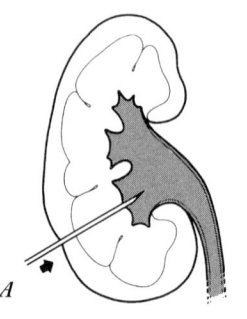
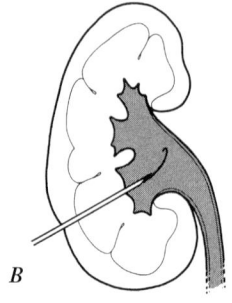
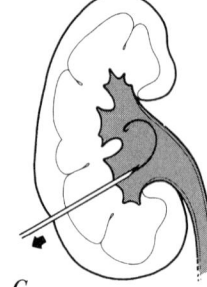

Fig. 11. The procedure used for percutaneous nephrostomy: (A) needle insertion, (B) passage of a guide wire, and (C) passage of the catheter.

Drainage Catheters

Amplatz became involved in the development of balloon-less, self-retaining drainage catheters in the early 1980s. In cooperation with Tadavarthy in 1984, Amplatz developed a dual-stiffness Malecot, self-retaining drainage catheter (Figure 12A). The

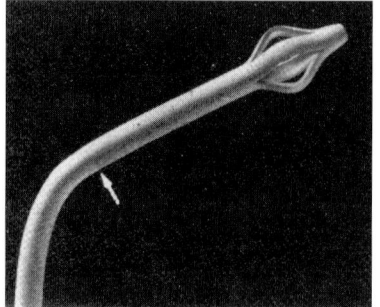
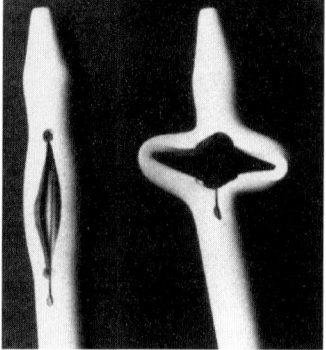

Fig. 12. A dual stiffness catheter (A) shown with the juncture of two plastics of different stiffness (arrow) and a dual stiffness, self-retaining drainage catheter (B) with internal monofilament for expanding the tip.

catheter was created for drainage of the urinary bladder, gallbladder, or a pus-filled cavity. A major disadvantage of previous drainage catheters was their stiffness, which resulted in patient discomfort. The new catheter had a stiff tip, made by slitting the catheter longitudinally and heat forming it in the expanded position. The tip was straightened by the force of a flexible stiffener within the catheter. Both catheter and stiffener were advanced over a wire guide into the desired cavity; the stiffener was then removed, allowing the catheter to resume its original shape, which provided retention.

In collaboration with Smith, Amplatz developed another type of retention-drainage catheter in 1986. As shown in Figure 12B, the tip was closed and opened by tension applied to a nylon monofilament, which was affixed to the inside of the tip and connected to a locking device at the proximal end. After placing the catheter (containing a stiffener) over a wire guide in the cavity to be drained, Amplatz and Smith withdrew the wire guide and stiffener and operated the locking apparatus to place tension on the monofilament, which expanded the winged tip.

Because it is customary to affix a stopcock to self-retaining drainage catheters, Amplatz devised a way to combine the stopcock motion with that employed to expand the catheter tip.

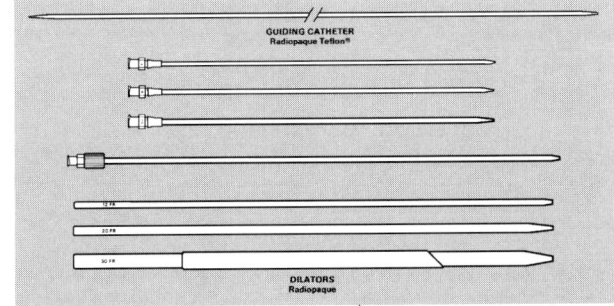

Fig. 13. The Amplatz renal dilator set and its components.

Using the Nephrostomy Tract for Other Purposes

While the nephrostomy tract was first used for drainage, it soon became apparent that the tract could also be used for stone removal and stent implantation. When used for stone removal, the tract must be larger than the diameter of the largest stone to be removed, so Rusnak and Amplatz in 1982 developed a set of coaxial dilating Teflon catheters (Figure 13). By passing successively larger-diameter catheters, the nephrostomy tract could be dilated to the desired size, thereby allowing removal of large stones and the insertion of nephroscopes.

Early steps in percutaneous nephrostomy were taken by Fernström in 1976 and by Smith in 1979. Smith and his colleagues reported using the nephrostomy tract to dissolve renal and ureteral stones, or to remove them with a basket catheter or forceps.

Removing Urinary Stones

In 1982, Castaneda-Zuniga and Amplatz described the basic technique for urinary stone removal. First they visualized the upper urinary system by injecting contrast medium through a small bore needle. Then they punctured a posterior calix and created and dilated the nephrostomy tract to the desired diameter, which was typically 30 French but could be as large as 50 French. Under fluoroscopic guidance, they identified and extracted the stones with Randall forceps or a Dormia basket at the tip of a catheter. (The Dormia basket was first described by

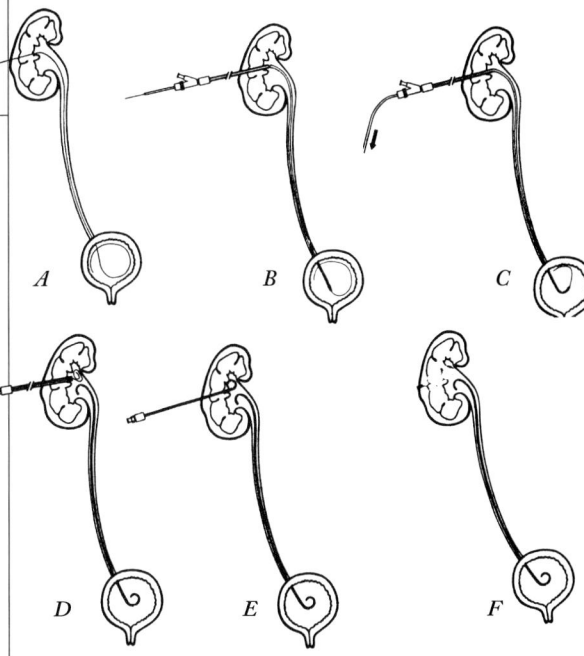

Fig. 14. To place the Amplatz ureteral stent, a guide wire was placed into the bladder percutaneously through a needle (A), the stent was advanced over the guide wire with the stent introducer (B), the guide wire was withdrawn (C, D), the introducer was withdrawn (E), and the double-J stent was in place (F).

Lagrave in 1969, who used it to extract biliary stones through a Kehr drainage tube.)

Many influential papers on percutaneous stone removal subsequently came out of Amplatz's laboratory. In a review of the experience at University of Minnesota, Coleman in 1985 stated that the success rate with percutaneous removal of stones had increased since the early 1980s to 99% in a study of 450 patients. This high success rate was largely due to the tools and techniques developed by Amplatz and to his close collaboration with an experienced urology team.

In addition to drainage and stone removal, nephrostomy tracts were also used to place stents. In 1985, in collaboration with Cardella, Amplatz developed a double-stent catheter made of C-Flex, a soft plastic material. Figure 14 shows how the stent was inserted and resumed its double pigtail shape when the stiff wire guide was withdrawn.

Amplatz Vena Cava Filters

Many vena cava filters had been designed for percutaneous placement, but, until later, none could be removed percutaneously. Amplatz set forth the criteria for the ideal vena cava filter: It should filter thrombi, not obstruct flow, be nonthrombogenic and biocompatible, be placed percutaneously, not migrate after installation, not damage the surrounding tissue, and be retrievable percutaneously.

In 1984, Lund and Amplatz described such a device (Figure 15). It consisted of a spider-like structure that was screwed onto a wire introducer. The piercing wires were set by pulling back gently on the delivery wire. Then the filter was released by unscrewing the device. A loop at the other end allowed retrieval with a snare. The spider consisted of eighteen inert alloy wires. Each wire had a prong that pierced the vessel wall and a loop that limited penetration to 2 mm. The filter diameter was 12 mm in the first animal studies and 28 mm in human trials. Although studied extensively, this filter was never made commercially available.

Nitinol Stents

Like Dotter, Amplatz became interested in using the metallic alloy nitinol—the metal with a thermal memory—to create an arterial stent. This alloy can be shaped into a desired form at elevated temperatures. When cooled, it straightens. Then, when exposed to 37°C blood, it reverts to its shaped form.

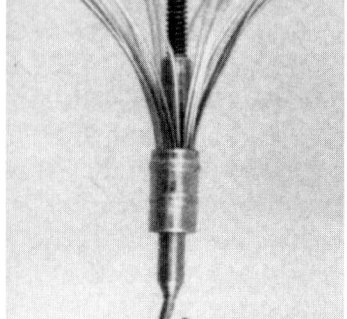
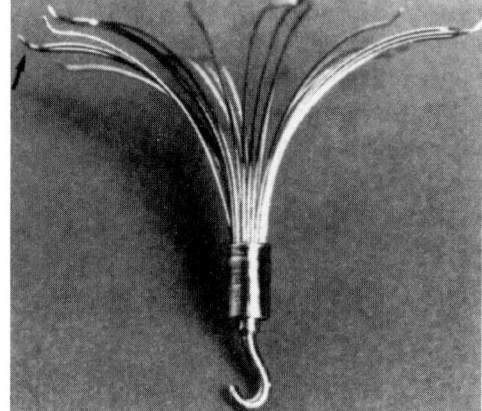

A B

Fig. 15. Two views of the Amplatz percutaneously insertable and removable vena cava filter. The top arrow in (A) identifies the threaded part that engages with the delivery wire. In (B), at the bottom is the loop snared for removal.

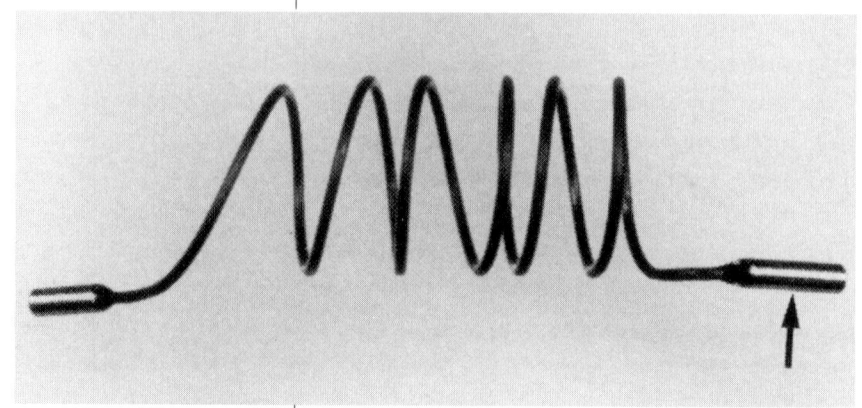

Fig. 16. At the ends of this nitinol wire coil stent are adapters that couple to a guide wire.

In 1983, Cragg and Amplatz used 0.01-inch diameter nitinol wire to construct a series of coil stents for percutaneous insertion into a dog's abdominal aorta. The coils ranged from 5 to 11 mm in diameter and from 1 to 6 cm long. (Figure 16 is an example.) They were wound on mandrels and preformed at 525°C for thirty minutes. The stents were then chilled in ice water, straightened out, and introduced through a Teflon catheter inserted in the aorta. As the nitinol wire emerged from the catheter and came into contact with warm blood, it resumed its coil shape. The wire guide was then unscrewed and withdrawn with the catheter.

Cragg and Amplatz performed angiographic studies of the nitinol coil stents at one and four weeks after implantation into four dogs. Commenting on the results, they said that the coil acted like a conventional porous stent that functioned as a template for formation of a neointima.

Contributions to Balloon Dilation and Angioplasty

Balloon dilation of the prostate was described by Castaneda and Amplatz in many papers. In 1979, Castaneda and Amplatz summarized the centuries-old history of dilation of the prostatic urethra and described their latest human studies with a 25-mm diameter balloon, inflated with a pressure of 6 atmospheres (90 psi) for ten minutes. The pressure was readjusted during those ten minutes as the prostate dilated. In eight of nine patients, the dilation increased the ease of urine flow. Castaneda and Amplatz pointed out that the procedure could be performed on outpatients, without general anesthesia.

While many investigators experimented with new techniques and discovered that they were effective, Amplatz and his associates were among the first to investigate the reasons why these techniques worked. For example, after Dotter and Judkins introduced percutaneous arterial angioplasty in the early 1960s, the mechanism of the procedure was thought to be the redistribution and compression of atheromatous material in the vessel. Amplatz and his colleagues (Castaneda-Zuniga in 1980–1981 and Zollikofer in 1984) investigated these mechanisms, challenged this classic concept, and advanced a new theory based on animal and cadaver studies. Castaneda-Zuniga et al observed that, as solids and semiliquids, atheromatous plaques were incompressible. Therefore, balloon inflation in the vessel resulted in cracking of the intima and pulling away of this intimal layer from the media. The artery wall itself literally stretched from the balloon's pressure and remained open by the blood pressure. Healing of the disrupted arterial layers occurred by the formation of a neointima and scar tissue.

Assessing Vascular Damage

Many researchers have studied the effects of balloon angioplasty. Zollikofer et al, for example, demonstrated that soon after balloon angioplasty, intimal walls were stripped and widespread deterioration of muscle cells and rupture of collagen fibers occurred. After two weeks, reendothelialization occurred and there was evidence of intimal growth. Dilated arterial segments were repaired by proliferation of myocytes and collagen and intima formation. Two to three months later, intima and media repair was complete. After six months, dilated segments were characterized by continued intimal growth and increased media collagen content.

Amplatz and his colleagues stated that the degree of vascular damage following dilation was related to balloon size, duration of pressure, and number of inflations. After the healing process, long-lasting patency was expected. However, they wrote, "Whether or not intimal hyperplasia occurs with the same frequency in normal and atherosclerotic vessels is not known. If the same mechanism occurs, it may be beneficial to put a patient on a low-cholesterol diet after percutaneous transluminal angioplasty to minimize risk factors until the reendothelialization is established."

Scientific Apparatus Shop

The Scientific Apparatus Shop at the University of Minnesota was founded in 1921 to assist the entire faculty with a support staff of skilled technicians. It was in this shop that the creative ideas of Amplatz and his colleagues became hardware, and consequently they did not rely on manufacturers for the design and production of new equipment. Today, the shop has several full-time employees and is equipped with lathes, milling machines, drill presses, welding equipment, and sheet metal-working equipment. The apparatus group is funded by the State of Minnesota to defray some of the expenses of research that requires experimental work.

When Amplatz joined the university, the shop was under the direction of Larry Espy, a highly trained experimental machinist who is now retired. Amplatz also worked closely with Frank Kotula for thirty years. Although Kotula is also now retired from the shop staff, he still works part-time. He built the first heart-lung machine and numerous heart valves, as well as all the devices designed by Amplatz and his colleagues.

About Amplatz

Kurt Amplatz was born in 1924 in Senftenberg, a village of about one thousand residents in lower Austria. His father was a physician in general medical practice in Senftenberg and in Misslitz, Czechoslovakia. Amplatz was a soccer player,

THE AMPLATZ-COOK PARTNERSHIP

Kurt Amplatz has used his scientific curiosity to create a variety of devices. His work with Cook Incorporated has produced the following products, which have been widely used in urology and interventional radiology:

- BH (benzalkonium heparin) coating for wire guides
- Amplatz Extra Stiff Wire Guide
- Soft Shaft Malecot Catheter
- Amplatz Retention Catheter
- Amplatz Renal Dilator Set
- Amplatz Ureteral Stent Set

These devices, combined with Amplatz's extensive writing and teaching, have helped set the course for radiology as the field enters its second century.

---

swimmer, and fencer while in high school in Innsbruck, but his favorite pastime was experimenting in the chemistry laboratory at the university where his uncle was a professor. World War II was in full force, and he remembers the constant bombings, shattered glass, and lack of heat and running water. There was only one functioning toilet in his neighborhood, and it was necessary to arrive at 5:00 a.m. to wait in line. He recalls having difficulty with studying and memorizing, attributing it to poor food rations that consisted mainly of cabbage. While writing his final exam (in Italian) there was an air raid.

Following the war, Amplatz attended the University of Innsbruck, where he received his medical degree in 1951. Although Austria was under Russian occupation, he was able to obtain additional medical training in Fribourg and Zurich, Switzerland, and Paris, France. He served an internship in Austria, and then he came to the United States and interned at St. Johns Hospital, Brooklyn, New York.

Amplatz applied for a residency at the Mayo Clinic but was not accepted. He was, however, accepted for residency training at Receiving Hospital at Wayne State University in Detroit, where he remained from 1954 to 1957. After completing training in radiology, he joined the University of Minnesota as an instructor. He sought this appointment because of the outstanding research reputation of the x-ray department, then headed by Leo Rigler. Amplatz became an assistant professor of radiology in 1961, associate professor in 1963, and full professor in 1970.

Amplatz is at present interested in writing books and working on scientific papers with his colleagues. To date he has trained more than one hundred fellows who have carried the Amplatz spirit of adventure with them around the world.

Amplatz is not all business—he enjoys windsurfing, skiing, and playing tennis. A private man, he has four children and a black Labrador retriever, which he predicted would be as well trained as his fellows in radiology.

Publications and Awards

Amplatz began publishing while an instructor in radiology at the University of Minnesota. By the early 1990s he had published 557 papers (with an additional 30 submitted and 29 in press at the time of this writing), 6 books (of which he was the senior author on 2), 33 book chapters, 17 abstracts, 151 conference papers, and 17 scientific exhibits.

Although Amplatz is best known for publications in angiography, angioplasty, and endourology, his first paper (in 1958) dealt with the use of air as a contrast medium to visualize the stomach and duodenum. A period followed in which he reported many improvements in angiographic equipment and techniques; then his many publications appeared on congenital and acquired cardiovascular abnormalities, angioplasty, and urology.

Published Six Books

Amplatz has published six books: *Congenital Heart Disease* (1971), *Coronary Angiography* (1973), *Clinical Angiographic and Pathology Profiles* (1976), *Cardiovascular Radiology* (1984), *Atlas of Endourology* (1986), and *Radiology of Congenital Heart Disease* (1986).

Radiology of Congenital Heart Disease reflects Amplatz's early and continuing interest in this subject. The book covers cardiac anatomy and defects, outflow obstructions, cardiac catheterization, angiography, x-ray equipment (including image intensifiers and videotape recording), film properties, radiation safety, and electrical hazards. It contains the following statement: "Finally we hope that currently in our environment there is the germ of an idea, or the development of a new collaborative effort which will result in new ideas and better volumes to replace this work. Then our work as teachers will be complete."

Amplatz received the Magna Cum Laude award in 1980 from the Radiological Society of North America (RSNA) for his scientific exhibit on the mechanics of angioplasty. For the same research, the Canadian Association of Radiologists awarded him First Prize in 1981 and the American Roentgen Ray Society (ARRS) granted him its Certificate of Merit. The RSNA also awarded him the Certificate of Merit for his research on transluminal angioplasty.

Amplatz's scientific exhibit on the percutaneous removal of renal stones received an ARRS gold medal and the RSNA Cum Laude citation. A scientific report by Coleman and Amplatz on stone removal was recognized in 1985 by the *American Journal of Radiology* as one of the most important papers on the subject. In 1988, Amplatz was Gold Medalist at the American College of Radiology meeting and received the Memorial Award from the Chicago Radiological Society. The New York Academy of Medicine recognized him with the 29th Ferdinand C. Valentine Award. For his scientific exhibit on percutaneous ureteral clipping, the RSNA awarded him the Certificate of Merit.

He that invents a
machine augments
the power of a man
and the well-being
of mankind.

Henry Ward Beecher

CHAPTER 9: Cesare Gianturco

The Giant of Coils, Filters, and Stents

For more than sixty years, Cesare Gianturco's creative imagination has given rise to a wide variety of original interventional techniques and devices, including the cotton-tail embolus, wool coils, the Bird's Nest filter, expandable stents, and the first balloon catheter.

Near the beginning of his career, in 1933, Gianturco developed devices in association with John Camp at the Mayo Clinic that facilitated radiographic examination of the optic and hypoglossal canals, determined the proper position of calcified pineal glands, and allowed direct measurement of the diameter of the pelvis.

The previous year, in 1932, he had collaborated with Walter Alvarez at the Mayo Clinic in the pioneering use of early cineradiographic surgical techniques to study hunger contractions in cat stomachs. He later used the same techniques to study the mechanics of the pyloric-duodenal area and then, with Kirklin, to examine gallbladder contractions without using contrast material. In 1934, working with Leddy, Desjardins, and Counsellor, he determined the effects of radiation therapy on bone metastases from prostatic carcinoma.

Throughout his career, Gianturco's keen mind has been able to meet diagnostic and therapeutic challenges in new ways. He joined the staff of the Carle Clinic in Champaign, Illinois, in 1934 to work in clinical radiology. While at the clinic, he developed techniques to improve bronchograms and used high-voltage radiography for colon examinations. He was able to combine routine clinical radiography with proctoscopy and at the same time obtain laboratory specimens to save clinic patients time and discomfort.

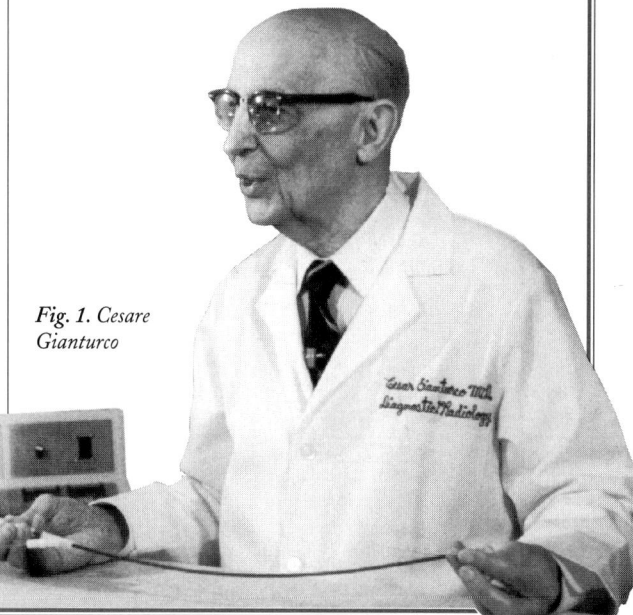

Fig. 1. Cesare Gianturco

Wartime Innovations

During World War II, Gianturco served in the U.S. Army Medical Corps in the United States and Europe. His contributions to the war effort were a stereoscopic method of localizing metallic foreign bodies in the eye and a technique to determine retinal damage by passing a flat, thin x-ray beam through injured eyes.

After World War II, he returned to the Carle Clinic and remained there until his retirement in 1968. However, perhaps the most productive years of Gianturco's scientific life have come in the more than twenty years since his official retirement. After his retirement and a brief hiatus, he joined the diagnostic radiology department at The University of Texas M.D. Anderson Hospital and Tumor Institute at Houston. Shortly after Gianturco arrived at Anderson, John S. Dunn, Sr., financed an experimental diagnostic laboratory there that was later also supported by William Cook, president of Cook Incorporated.

While in Houston, Gianturco, along with Wallace, Anderson, and others, designed an experiment to determine the best dosage of heparin to be administered just before interventional radiologic vascular procedures. He also designed, with the help of Tom Osborne and the Cook Incorporated research and development department, a pulsatile pump that delivered chemotherapeutic drugs in a pulsitile fashion into the blood. Later, in response to requests from the radiology staff, Gianturco, Anderson, and Wallace developed two new types of embolizing devices and the tapered catheters used for their delivery.

Embolizing Devices

Gianturco was not the first investigator to achieve embolization through a catheter. Others researchers had placed embolization materials percutaneously into appropriate vessels to treat arteriovenous malformations, gastrointestinal bleeding, neoplasms of the uterus and kidney, epistaxis, and other conditions, but the materials they used resulted in varying degrees of success.

Gianturco and his associates sought new materials that were safe, permanent, and easily introduced into the vessel of choice. In 1975, Gianturco, Anderson, and Wallace described two original devices that they dubbed "cotton tails" and "wool coils." They used the cotton tails in small arteries and the wool coils in larger arteries.

Cotton Tails and Wool Coils

The cotton tails were emboli that consisted of eight strands of cotton thread 5 mm long attached to the end of a 3-mm segment of 19-gauge steel tubing (Figure 2). Gianturco inserted a 6-French polyethylene catheter into the exposed femoral arteries of dogs and advanced it to the site to be embolized. He then impaled the fabricated cotton-tail embolus on the centrally tapered mandrel of a 20-gauge Karras needle and inserted the needle into the catheter. When the catheter was properly positioned, Gianturco withdrew the needle and mandrel, leaving the cotton tail in the catheter lumen. He then injected the

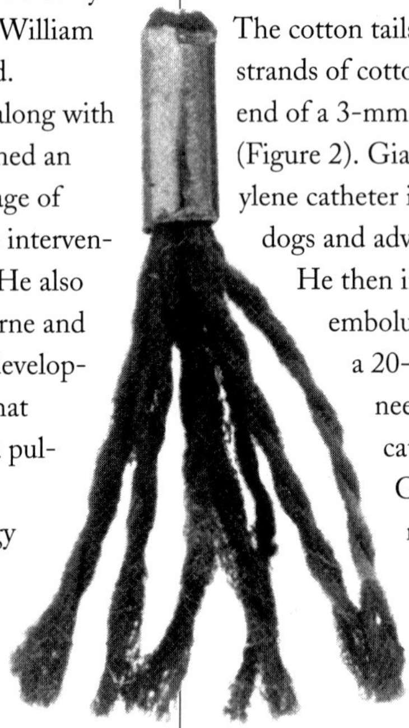

Fig. 2. The cotton-tail embolus consisting of eight cotton strands, 5 mm long, attached to a 3-mm segment of 19-gauge steel tubing.

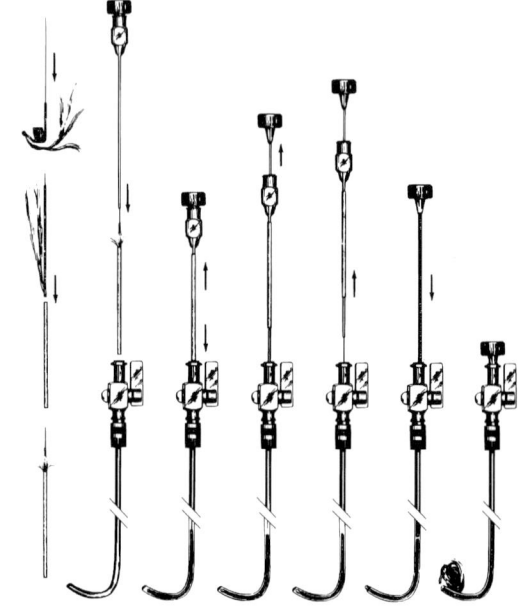

Fig. 3. Technique for placement of embolizing wool coils.

cotton tail into the vessel with a bolus of saline and withdrew the catheter. Blood flow took the embolus into a small artery 2 mm or less in diameter until it wedged in the artery or ran into a bifurcation. Gianturco used this technique to occlude coronary, renal, celiac, and mesenteric arteries in dogs.

To occlude larger arteries, Gianturco and his associates attached four woolen strands, each 3 cm long, to one end of a tightly coiled 5 cm long segment of steel guide wire that had its central core removed. The researchers straightened the coiled guide wire with an introducer, which consisted of a fine-wire mandrel protruding from a long piece of 19-gauge steel tubing. The tubing fit inside a previously positioned 7-French Teflon catheter and was long enough to deposit the wool coil near the terminal curve of the catheter (Figure 3). After they withdrew the introducer, Gianturco and his associates pushed the coil into the arterial lumen with a modified 0.045 inch guide wire. When released into the artery, the wool coil regained its original coiled shape and formed an embolus of steel and wool.

The researchers found the wool coils and cotton-tail emboli to be superior to any embolic materials previously used, such as autologous clots, Gelfoam, stainless steel wire, and subcutaneous tissue. Autologous clots were subject to lysis and lasted only a few days, and Gelfoam did not always result in occlusion. Pieces of stainless steel wire (without cotton threads attached) acquired a thin covering of fibrin, came to equilibrium in the artery, and lost their effectiveness to occlude. Subcutaneous tissue was in scarce supply.

Clinical Trials

Satisfied with trials in dogs that showed persistent arterial occlusion two weeks after they placed the wool coils, Gianturco and his associates successfully used the coils to occlude the renal arteries of two patients with hypernephromas. They achieved subsequent success in patients with renal carcinomas, renal arteriovenous fistulas, hepatic carcinomas, hypersplenism, and giant-cell tumors of the sacrum. They were able to use the wool coils to occlude renal veins as well as renal, hepatic, splenic, and internal iliac arteries.

Arterial embolization facilitated surgery by reducing tumor vascularity, and it was found to be useful for palliative debulking of inoperable tumors. Two coils were usually used for vascular occlusion, but as many as five coils might be needed to obtain satisfactory results.

Gianturco, Anderson, and Wallace investigated the coil's ability to occlude arteriovenous fistulas in dogs by constructing a vascular conduit to connect the common carotid artery and external jugular vein. Occluding arteriovenous fistulas with particulate embolic material presented the danger of the occluding substances being swept into venous circulation and then into the pulmonary vasculature.

Gianturco and his colleagues determined the importance of two features of their device: coil size and the presence of wool strands. If the coil was too large for the fistula, it had a tendency to unwind and protrude beyond the fistula; wool strands promoted clot formation. The physicians observed that if they placed a coil without strands into an artery or vein, the vessel was still patent one hour after coil placement. In contrast, when they placed a coil with wool strands, complete occlusion occurred within five minutes. Using several coils without wool strands, however, was effective in obstructing large diameter, high-flow arteries quickly. In small diameter arteries that were able to accommodate only a single coil, the wool strands hastened clot formation.

By 1979, wool coils were being referred to as "Gianturco coils," and Dacron was used in addition to or in place of wool strands because some interventional radiologists objected to the use of wool. They perceived that wool could not be sterilized by steam, a method preferred by many to sterilization by gas. (Wool sometimes carries tetanus spores not neutralized by steam.) Gianturco believed that wool was better than Dacron and could be effectively sterilized by gas methods.

The Mini-Coil

Gianturco also developed a smaller version of the wool coil, called the "mini" coil. One of the earliest uses of a steel mini-coil was in a twelve-year-old girl with a giant-cell tumor of the fourth lumbar vertebra. She was unable to walk despite having received chemotherapy and cobalt treatments. Arteriography indicated that the blood supply to the tumor originated from several lumbar arteries. Gianturco selectively catheterized these arteries using a 5-French polyethylene catheter, injected Gelfoam cubes to interrupt blood flow to the tumor, and inserted mini-coils into the lumbar arteries to ensure occlusion and prevent recanalization. Five weeks later, the patient was ambulatory and the lesion was considerably smaller than before the embolization procedure.

The mini-coil offered several advantages over its larger predecessor. First, it had a tighter, more secure fit in small vessels. Standard coils tended to elongate when placed in small diameter vessels, protruding beyond the ends of the vessel targeted for embolization and extending into the aorta. Elongation also compromised the thrombogenic effectiveness of the coil.

A second advantage of the mini-coil was that it could be inserted through a 5-French polyethylene catheter. The catheter's small size and flexibility permitted greater selectivity in catheterization procedures. Mini-coils were best for vessels with a diameter ranging from two to four millimeters, while standard size coils were better suited for larger structures.

Gianturco first used catheters with untapered tips to place the coils. He eventually modified a third-generation Gianturco coil so that it could be introduced through a tapered-tip catheter, thus simplifying the placement procedure. In later versions, shorter Dacron strands were placed along the length of the wire coil rather than attached to the end. This axial placement of strands gave the modified coil the appearance of a fuzzy caterpillar (Figure 4) and allowed the coil to be inserted through a tapered-tip catheter.

Gianturco and his associates were not the first ones to occlude arteries selectively to control bleeding, to treat arteriovenous malformations, or to reduce blood flow to carcinomas. However, they did make important contributions to these procedures, including the introduction of new occluding devices, the refinement of device design, and the development of a variety of applications.

Bird's Nest Filters

Decades before Gianturco's first paper on vascular filters was published, various devices had been used to protect the pulmonary vasculature from emboli. However, there were problems associated with the devices and many investigators were seeking safer and more effective methods.

In a 1980 paper, Gianturco identified the main attributes of a good vena cava filter:
- The filter should be small enough to be inserted percutaneously through a small catheter.

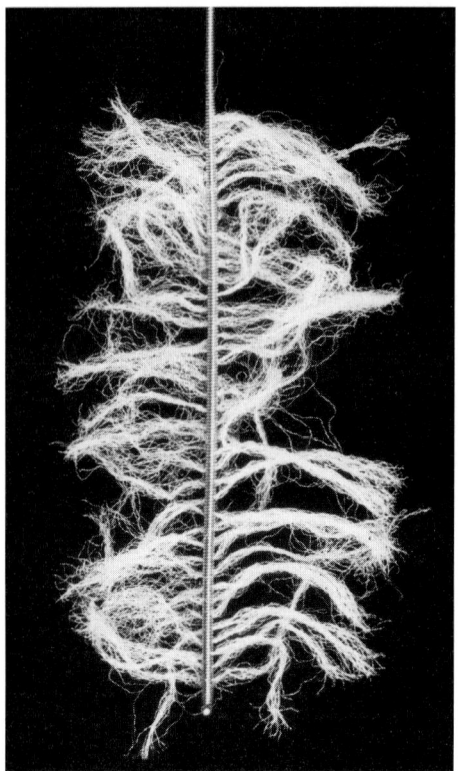

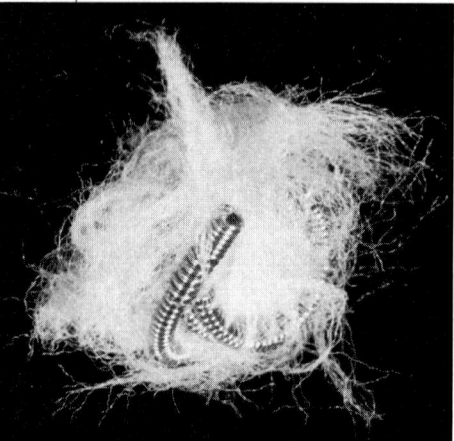

Fig. 4. The occluding spring embolus catheter. (A) When extended, the embolus looked like a "fuzzy caterpillar." (B) The coiled device was an effective occluder.

Fig. 5. This prototype was a forerunner of the Bird's Nest filter.

- It should be short enough to be placed in the vena cava below the renal veins and above the iliac veins.
- It should have minimal surface area exposed to blood flow so that it does not obstruct the flow.
- It should not be an additional source of emboli.
- It should be securely anchored to the vena cava so that it will not migrate.

The First Prototype

With these criteria, Gianturco and his associates fabricated the first prototype of a vena cava filter using three very fine stainless steel wires (0.010 mm in diameter) about as thick as a human hair. The wires were shaped into nonmatching curves and tied together at their ends, forming a tangled web designed to trap migrating emboli. One end of the nest-like filter was attached to a long, straight wire that was fixed beneath the skin of the groin. The three wires needed to be straightened to be inserted into a catheter, but the bends of the wires would reform after the catheter was withdrawn when it was in the desired position (Figure 5).

Fig. 6. Vena cava and filter removed from a dog four weeks after placement. Note areas of intimal proliferation (arrows) where filter wires contacted the vessel walls.

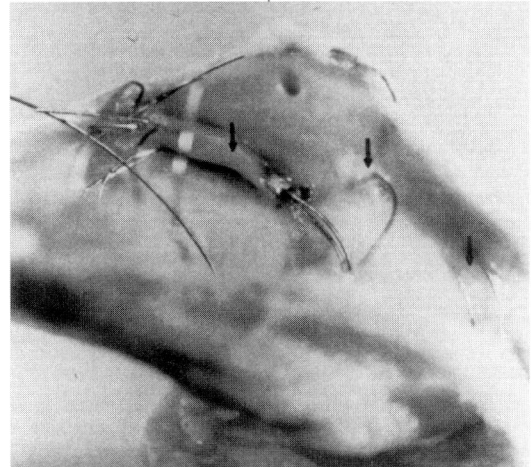

Using fluoroscopy, Gianturco placed the filters into the venae cavae of eighteen anesthetized dogs through a 6.5-French catheter inserted via an exposed right femoral vein. The filters were positioned midway between the renal veins and the iliac bifurcation. The dogs were sacrificed at three days and at one, two, four, six, and eight weeks after filter placement. None of the dogs demonstrated vena caval obstruction or thrombi on the wire struts of the filters. Gianturco postulated that the small surface area of the wires deterred clotting. At the points where the thin wires contacted the intima, tissue surrounded them and fixed the filter in position, preventing migration (Figure 6).

Fig. 7. The original vena cava filter was anchored with a tin sphere embedded into subcutaneous groin tissue.

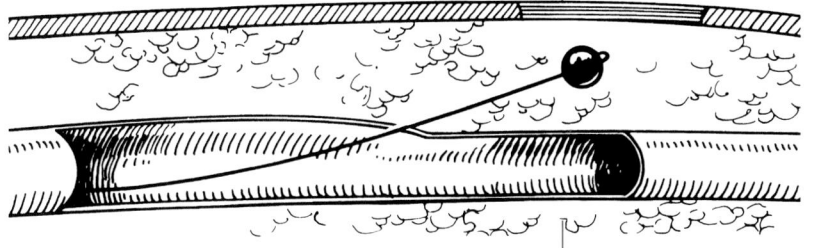

A Second Prototype

After repeated modifications of the filter following tests in animals, Gianturco developed a second prototype, which had four bent wires instead of three, providing a tighter filtering mesh. Clinical trials of this filter began in 1982. In 1984, Roehm suggested a different anchoring system to Gianturco. Originally, the proximal end of the straight wire that carried the filter was formed into a curve and attached to a split tin sphere. The tin sphere was then anchored in the subcutaneous tissue of the groin (Figure 7). In the newer model, the anchoring system was comprised of a special set of two prongs attached to both ends of the filter. Each prong had a double hook and a flexible stop so that it would not enter too far after penetrating the wall of the vein. In his 1984 paper, Roehm referred to the device as a "bird's nest" filter, its popular designation and now a trademark name.

A most attractive feature of the Bird's Nest filter is its ability to be placed percutaneously, eliminating the need for laparotomy. The Bird's Nest filter, however, lacks retrievability. Gianturco feels that since the intima grows over the wire in two weeks, any attempt to retrieve the filter could easily tear a vein and is not worth the risk.

The Bird's Nest filter has been placed in thousands of patients and has performed well. Recurrent pulmonary thromboemboli were suspected clinically in 2.7% of patients, and vena caval occlusion in 2.9% of patients. According to Roehm et al (1988), the modified fixation mechanism is sound and filter migration has not been reported. Katsamouris et al reported in 1988 that when compared to a variety of other in vitro circulation filters, the Bird's Nest filter wins high marks for its ability to trap clots, regardless of configurational orientation, and for its relative lack of negative effects on blood flow dynamics.

Zigzag Stents and the Balloon Catheter Stent

In 1969, long before Gianturco began experimenting with stents, Dotter reported transluminal placement of intraluminal devices to enlarge vessels narrowed by atheromatous plaque. Dotter placed tubular prostheses (usually introduced through the left carotid artery) into normal femoral and popliteal arteries of twenty-five dogs. The impervious tubular grafts occluded within twenty-four hours, a patency period clearly too short for any clinical application.

Dotter then substituted tubular prostheses fabricated in the form of coil springs rather than impervious plastic tubes and reported that two out of three uncoated coil prostheses were still patent more than two years after placement, demonstrating the feasibility of successful intraluminal stenting.

Z Stents Developed

In 1985, Gianturco and his associates (Wright et al) described an expandable stent made of bare stainless steel wire 0.018 mm in diameter. The wire was bent six to eight times in opposite directions, and the ends were joined together to form a cylinder. These zigzag or Z stents were compressed to fit in the lumen of a catheter and then pushed out of the catheter with a flat-ended pusher (Figure 8). When they left the catheter, the stents reexpanded to dilate the vessel.

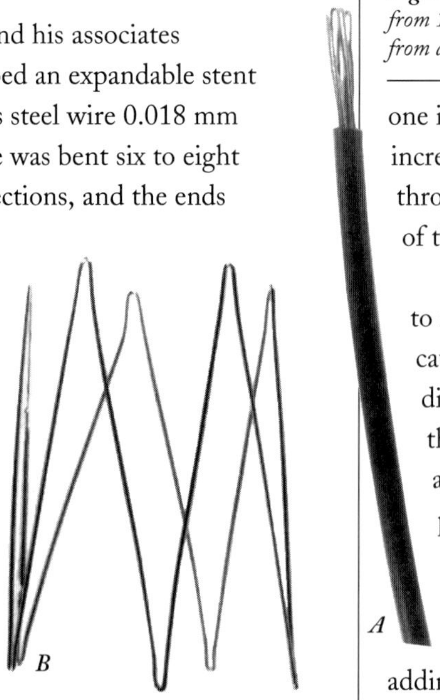

Gianturco's zigzag stents were passed into the jugular vein, abdominal aorta, and vena cava of dogs. Six months after placement there were no flow defects, narrowing, or occlusion. Furthermore, no agent was required to induce the stent to conform to the diameter of the vessel, and side branches that were crossed by stent wires remained patent. Because the fully expanded stents were somewhat larger than the vessel's diameter, migration was minimal. Within two to three weeks after placement, the stent wires were encased by neointima, where they made contact with vessel walls.

Percutaneous placement was an attractive feature of Gianturco's stents. The expansile capability of the stents was determined by the diameter of the wire used, the angle of the bends, and the number of bends. Several stents could be layered, one inside another, with their ends overlapping to increase the stent's length. The stents were not thrombogenic; no clot formation was observed in any of the arteries that contained them.

Gianturco originally used the bare Z stents to relieve upper or lower vena cava obstructions caused by extensive growth or scarring. When he discovered that single Z stents could jump out of the catheter, Gianturco built double stents to avoid the jump. He also found that patients with some types of obstructions of the vena cava were not completely opened by two stents, and these patients could be helped by adding more stents placed inside previous ones. These additional stents had to be placed accurately; they were positioned by screwing the stretched end of a large guide wire to one of the Z bends and using the guide wire as a pusher. The guide wire was unscrewed after the additional stents were in position.

As Gianturco and his associates gained experience, they found that some obstructions were long enough to require a line of several stents. The stents could be kept in position and made somewhat flexible by using straight wire struts or by passing suture material through eyelets made at the bends, a technique devised by Uchida and Rösch.

Gianturco also tried the bare wire stents for intraluminal tumors, but the tumors kept growing between the wires. Rösch covered the bare stents with silicone material while Wright and Gianturco covered them with siliconized Dacron fabric. Both techniques enabled the Z stents to obstruct the growth of intraluminal tumors for a while.

The characteristic rigidity that results from the use of multiple Z stents, covered or bare, precludes their use in a small tortuous artery, especially if the artery is subject to continuous motion because of its anatomical location.

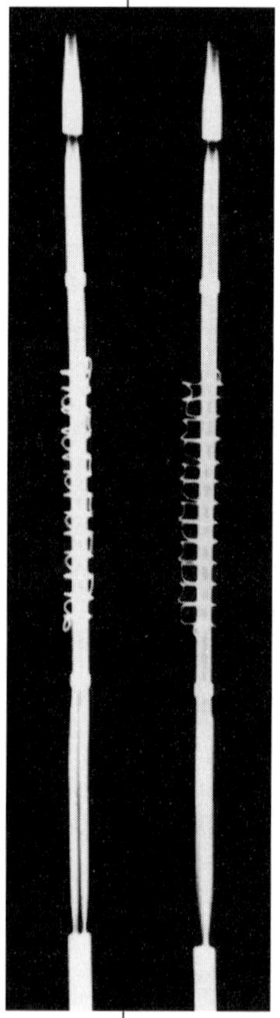

Balloon Catheter Stent for Coronary Arteries

Shortly before his death in 1985, Andreas Gruentzig asked Gianturco to design and build a stent for coronary arteries. The stent had to be quite small to negotiate the many bends of the coronary arteries. Gruentzig felt such a device could prevent restenosis. Gianturco and Roubin eventually devised a stent that was mounted directly on a balloon catheter and was expanded by inflating the balloon (Figure 9). After the stent expanded, the balloon was emptied and the catheter withdrawn. More than eight hundred patients have received flexible coronary stents to restore coronary patency after angioplasty relieves the stenosis. The same flexible stents could be used as stenotic arteriovenous dialysis stents.

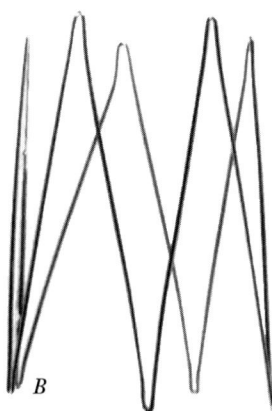

Fig. 8. Expandable stent. (A) End of collapsed stent emerging from 12-French sheath. (B) Fully expanded stent after release from delivery sheath.

Fig. 9. A balloon-expanded stainless steel stent. (A) reveals the angioplasty balloon-stent in the collapsed state. (B) shows the stent after inflation.

In 1985, Charnsangavej et al used segments of thoracic and abdominal aorta from human cadavers to model dissecting aneurysms. Two to three milliliters of contrast medium (30% meglumine diatrizoate) or normal saline was injected under the intima of the aortic segments, causing the lumen to bulge. Endovascular stents were placed into these simulated dissecting aneurysms. The expanded stents collapsed the bulging intima and restored the aortic lumen to its original dimensions.

In 1986, Charnsangavej also reported the placement of Gianturco stents in two patients with vena caval stenoses. One patient had superior vena cava syndrome secondary to carcinoma of the trachea. Charnsangavej placed four stents into the patient's right innominate vein and superior vena cava, and the patient experienced immediate relief of symptoms. He placed a fifth stent into the trachea to prevent collapse, with each inspiration, of a myocutaneous graft that was necessitated by partial resection of the distal trachea. The stents relieved troublesome symptoms of the vena cava syndrome and prevented collapse of the tracheal graft with respiration during the remaining three weeks of the patient's life.

The other patient had retroperitoneal leiomyosarcoma and edema of the legs and abdomen and evidenced marked stenosis of the vena cava at the L-4 level as shown on inferior cavography. Charnsangavej placed three Gianturco stents across the stenosis, resulting in an immediate decrease in the pressure gradient across the stenosis. Edema in the legs disappeared and did not recur. One of the stents migrated into the right ventricle by the next day; however, no symptoms related to that stent developed. When the patient died five months later with progressive neoplastic disease, an autopsy revealed an inferior vena cava encased by tumor but maintained patent by the remaining stents. There was no clotting on the caval stents, and the stent that migrated into the ventricle had been covered by endocardium and was free of clots.

Used for Atherosclerosis

In 1987, Rollins et al reported that Gianturco zigzag stents were effective in atherosclerotic animal models. These researchers induced atherosclerosis in the aortas of six rabbits by feeding them an atherogenic diet and traumatizing the intima. They placed eighteen stents into the six rabbits and left them in place for eight weeks. The ratio of stented to unstented diameters was 1.2 to 1. Where the stents contacted the vessel wall, they became encased with neointima, but the area of the stents that bridged side vessels was free of intima, thrombus, and fibrin.

According to Rollins' 1987 report, vessel dilation with expandable stents was apparently different from dilation by angioplasty. Angioplasty was more likely to split the plaque while the self-expanding stents dilated the vessel by stretching and compressing the intima and the media. Histologic examination of the rabbit aortas indicated that the tissue response to Gianturco stents (which exerted a continuous, dynamic force) was different from tissue response to angioplasty and placement of a passive endoprosthesis.

Having successfully reestablished and maintained patency in occluded large vessels, Duprat et al in 1987 turned their attention to the possibility of stenting small vessels to maintain patency following angioplasty. Thirty-three expandable metallic Gianturco stents 3, 4 and 5 mm in diameter (when fully expanded) were placed into the superficial femoral, popliteal, cranial tibial, saphenous, cranial mesenteric, renal, common hepatic, and splenic arteries of seven dogs. No anticoagulants were administered and radiographs were obtained at regular intervals. The dogs were sacrificed after 4, 6, 10, 12, 14, 16, or 30 weeks, and the vessel segments containing the stents were examined.

The success rate was 100% with stents 4 and 5 mm in diameter and 54% with 3-mm stents. None of the stents migrated or perforated the vessel wall. All side vessels bridged by the stents were patent and had not narrowed. The relationship of stent diameter to lumen diameter, called the stent-to-artery ratio (SAR), was crucial. When the SAR exceeded 1.2, complications developed. These complications included thrombosis with or without recanalization, vessel spasm, and excessive intimal proliferation over the stent wires. An SAR of 1.2 or less, however, resulted in an angiographic success rate of 100%.

A New U-Bend Design

According to Duprat, one limitation of the zigzag, self-expanding Gianturco stent was lack of longitudinal flexibility, so Gianturco addressed this shortcoming with a new stent design. Surgical suture wire (0.006 inch) was wrapped around a collapsed angioplasty catheter (25 mm long and 2.5 mm in diameter at full inflation). The wire was wrapped into a cylindrical shape with alternating U-shaped bends every 360°, with one upright U-bend and one inverted U-bend per turn (Figure 10). When inflated in the desired location, the angioplasty balloon expanded the diameter of the stent. Deflating the balloon allowed the catheter to be withdrawn and the expanded stent to remain within the vessel. The alternating U-bends imparted longitudinal flexibility to the stent, allowing it to adapt to movement or torsion.

Duprat placed stents fabricated in the new U-bend design into anesthetized dogs through a carotid arteriotomy under fluoroscopic guidance. When the stents were properly located, the angioplasty balloon was inflated several times to assure good stent expansion. After Duprat applied negative pressure to the angioplasty balloon, he removed the catheter, leaving the expanded flexible stent in place.

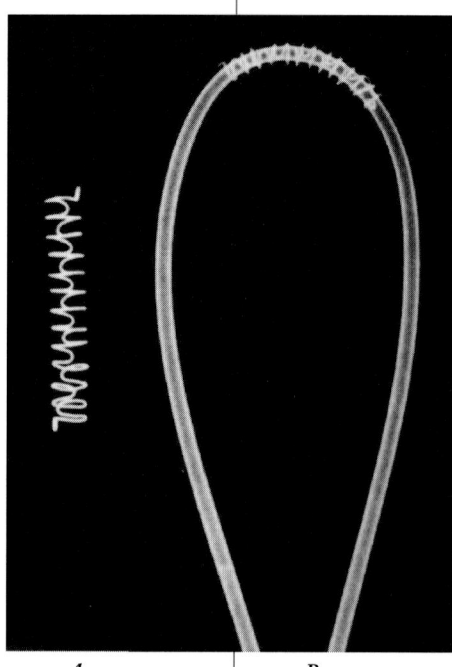

Fig. 10. Flexible balloon-expanded stent. (A) Expanded stent with balloon withdrawn showing alternating U-bends. (B) Demonstration of stent flexibility.

During a follow-up period of four to eight weeks, all the stents (which had been placed into the gluteal, saphenous, superficial femoral, or deep femoral artery) were patent. No stent migration occurred, and branching vessels covered by the stents remained patent, with only slight narrowing of a small branch bridged by a stent.

Although placement in coronary arteries was not described in the initial report of flexible stents, this application undoubtedly was anticipated and prompted Duprat to comment, "Flexibility is important if stents are to be inserted into small, continuously moving vessels with numerous curves and bends, such as the coronary arteries."

Placement of expandable Gianturco stents into nonvascular conduits was also a success. In 1986, Wallace et al successfully used expandable metal stents to buttress portions of the tracheobronchial tree. In 1985, Carrasco et al reported that placing Gianturco expansile stents into obstructed biliary ducts obviated the need for drainage catheters for decompression while relieving the obstruction. Because the stents are compressed during insertion, they could be placed percutaneously through a catheter as small as 8- or 9-French.

In 1988, Uchida et al used modified Gianturco stents with excellent results to treat patients with severe symptoms of superior vena cava syndrome. They also reported successful expansion of biliary stenoses in four patients with recurrent postsurgical tumorous stenoses. After demonstrating the feasibility of using expandable stents to relieve biliary obstruction, Uchida and associates modified the stents by adding flared skirts to increase their stability and prevent migration (Figure 11).

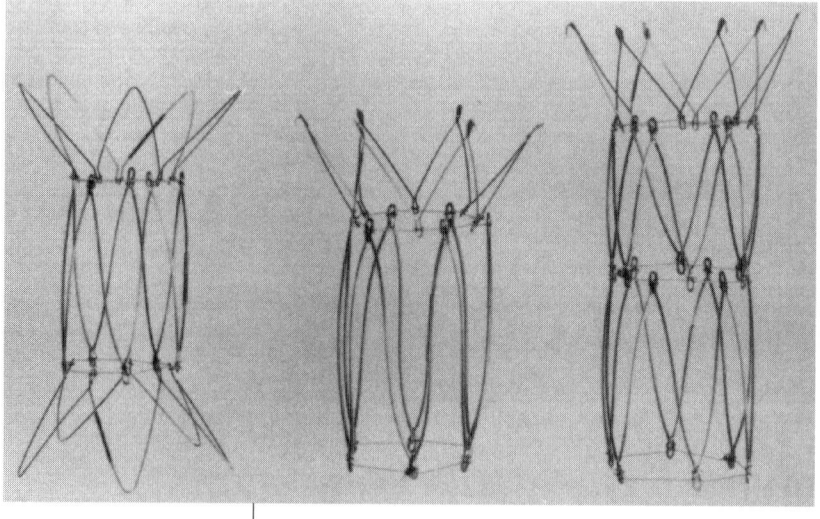

Fig. 11. Modified Gianturco expandable stents. (A) Double-skirted stent. (B) Single-skirted stent. (C) Single-skirted stent connected to a second nonmodified expandable stent.

Through his work with embolizing coils, vascular filters, and stents, Gianturco addressed the need to thrombose (with coils) certain vessels selectively, prevent embolization (with filters) in others, and reestablish patency (with stents) in yet others. Many scientists focus on only one or two questions throughout their careers. However, the sheer number and diversity of techniques and devices investigated and introduced by Cesare Gianturco make his contributions truly remarkable.

About Gianturco

Gianturco was born in Naples, Italy, in 1905, the youngest child in a family of eight children. His father was a lawyer who contributed much of his time and expertise to benefit Italy. He developed a set of standard regulations accepted by the mostly independent Italian city-states that aided those separate geopolitical entities in forming a unified country. Gianturco's father also served as the minister of transportation and was instrumental in building a railroad system linking remote parts of Italy.

Gianturco was not attracted to his father's public life, choosing instead a career in medicine. He entered the University of Naples, received a B.A. degree, and then completed his M.D. degree (cum laude) in 1927. After an internship in Naples, he served in the radiology residency program at the University of Rome from 1927 to 1929. From 1929 to 1930, he was a pathology resident at the University of Berlin, where he recalls learning to perform expedited autopsies. The technique involved removing all organs from the tongue to the rectum and arranging them on the examining table. The *oberprofessor* would then examine them and make his pronouncement.

Cineradiography Research

In 1930, Gianturco received a fellowship in surgery at the Mayo Clinic, where his brother was a surgeon. Tragically, two weeks after he arrived, his brother died. Gianturco then transferred to the radiology training program and served a four-year fellowship. His postgraduate work earned him a master of science degree in radiology, with a minor in physiology, from the University of Minnesota in 1933. While a fellow at the Mayo Clinic, with the support of his mentor Walter Alvarez, he began the task of determining if the empty stomach exhibited rhythmic contractions.

The motility of a stomach filled with contrast material had been demonstrated by Cannon soon after Roentgen introduced x-rays. The question remained, however, of how to determine radiographically whether or not an empty stomach is rhythmically active.

To answer that question, Gianturco developed one of the earliest cineradiographic systems ever made. First, he acquired a special 6-inch wide roll of film from Kodak. He then created a mechanism for advancing the film to obtain motion pictures of the fluoroscopic screen. To silhouette the stomach, he developed a method of inserting small lead pellets into the stomach wall along the greater curvature, with all pellets carefully placed in the same plane. Like Cannon (who introduced radiopaque barium to radiology), Gianturco used cats for his gastrointestinal studies because dogs were difficult to hold still. Female cats were more cooperative. He tried using a male cat once, but it escaped to the top of the x-ray machine and bit him when he tried to retrieve it.

Cineradiograms of the pellet-studded feline stomach showed that the empty stomach exhibited spontaneous contractions. Gianturco then proceeded to use the same lead-pellet technique to study motion of the pyloric duodenal region, again finding spontaneous contractions but at a higher rate than in the stomach and independent of gastric activity.

His Years at the Carle Clinic

In 1934, while still at the Mayo Clinic, Gianturco received an invitation to visit Vito Witting, a good friend and fellow immigrant from Italy. Witting knew Gianturco when both were residents at Mayo, before Witting left with several other Mayo doctors to help found the Carle Clinic in Champaign, Illinois. (Carle Clinic started as a tuberculosis sanitarium with land and funds

---

AND THE BEAT GOES ON

Cesare Gianturco remains active in his basement workshop in Champaign, Illinois. At present, he is working on a variety of ideas:

- Percutaneous closing of the ductus arteriosus and cardiac septal defects using fabric sacs filled with guide wire (with Wright).
- A percutaneous tubular prosthesis for establishing a central bypass in fusiform aneurysms of the abdominal aorta in elderly patients (with Wright and Guinn).
- Surgically implanted cardiac Dacron fabric disc valves.
- Reinforced Dacron discs for surgical repair of postoperative hernias of the abdominal wall (with Helfrich).

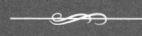

donated by the Carle family. However, it was not a financial success and was converted to a general medical service clinic.) Gianturco accepted Witting's invitation and arrived in Champaign the very day that Witting unexpectedly died from an undiagnosed case of acute leukemia.

While in Champaign and in shock from his friend's untimely death, Gianturco was offered the job that had been Witting's. He accepted the position and set about the task of building up the department of radiology. He also performed autopsies as part of his duties.

It was during his thirty-four years at the Carle Clinic that Gianturco developed his inventive skill for creating and perfecting new devices and procedures for interventional radiology. In the mid-1960s, for example, he came across a simple injector for lymphangiography that had been invented at Jefferson University Hospital in Philadelphia and that provided an alternative to the mechanical pump. A weight on the syringe plunger provided the force to push the plunger down, causing a steady stream of Lipiodol to flow out of the syringe, with the size of the syringe controlling the speed of injection. Gianturco improved the device and brought it to the attention of Cook Incorporated, which commercially developed the item for him just two weeks after he drew up his plans.

While at the Carle Clinic he met Verna Daily, who, although trained as an English teacher, was performing a number of duties at the clinic. They were married and raised two children.

Gianturco's interest in physiology continued and he devoted a half day each week on a voluntary basis to the physiology department of the University of Illinois at Urbana. The university showed its appreciation by appointing him clinical professor of physiology.

On to Anderson

In addition to his full-time position at the Carle Clinic and his commitment at the University of Illinois, Gianturco spent one day a week in Tuscola, Illinois, where the Carle Clinic operated a radiology department. In the middle of this hectic schedule, he was invited to join the research team at The University of Texas M.D. Anderson Hospital and Tumor Clinic at Houston. In 1968, when he retired from the Carle Clinic, he began spending six months a year at M.D. Anderson, where he organized an experimental radiology department with financial support from the Dunn Foundation and Cook Incorporated. This environment was tailor-made for Gianturco's creative genius because the hospital had animal research facilities and many patients in need of the kind of equipment that he loved to create.

Among the many devices Gianturco developed during this time was a pulsatile intermittent pump for the delivery of chemotherapeutic agents. Regular pumps usually provided a steady flow of agent, which could lead to a laminar flow inside the artery. The pulsatile pump, because it mixed the desired agent with the flow of blood, insured that an adequate amount of chemotherapeutic agent was delivered where it was needed.

In 1992, Cesare Gianturco was still going strong at the age of eighty-seven. He enjoys attending national conventions, where he can be seen holding court surrounded by interested physicians and technicians examining his latest device for interventional radiology. He remains incredibly productive, continuing to create ingenious percutaneously placed instruments. After sending prototypes to Tom Osborne of Cook Incorporated for production, he takes the devices to M.D. Anderson Hospital for tests in animals. When asked to explain his inability to stay away from developing new devices, he said, "I am a failure at retirement."

A Visit with Gianturco

While visiting Gianturco's home in Champaign, Illinois, we learned of his workshop museum in the basement (Figure 12). While we were there, he showed us such treasures from his workshop as a Marlex mesh for repairing hernias, vena cava filters, stents, a heart valve that can be delivered via a catheter, embolizing coils, a patent ductus occluder, a cystic duct occluder, and a subcutaneous access port.

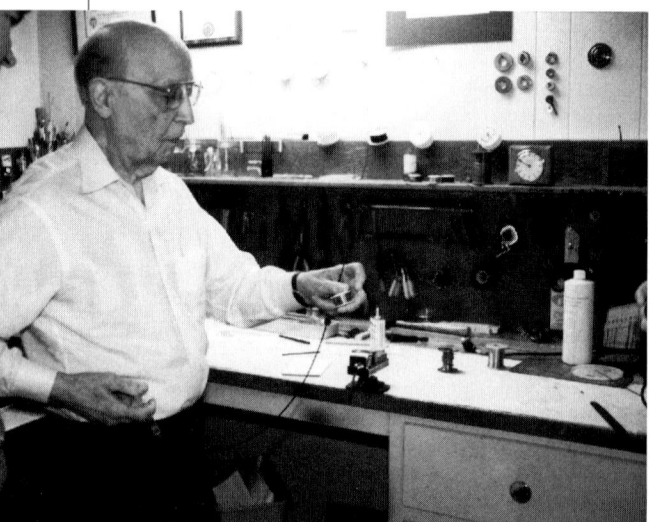

Fig. 12. Cesare Gianturco in his workshop.

He also showed us the first balloon dilation catheter that he designed, constructed, and used in the mid-1950s before Dotter, Porstmann, and Gruentzig devised their own balloon dilation catheters (Figure 13). The Gianturco dilator consisted of an 8-French catheter on which was mounted a 3-inch-long segment of polyolefin electrical shrink tubing. (The unshrunk part constituted the balloon.) The proximal and distal quarter-inch of the shrink tubing was shrunk (with the use of a heat gun obtained from Bill Cook) to embrace the catheter. In this pioneering device, the balloon was full size without inflation. When negative pressure was applied within the balloon, it shrunk, embracing the catheter and allowing it to be inserted. The balloon reexpanded with release of the negative pressure. Gianturco used this device to widen a stenosis in a femoral artery of one patient.

We asked Gianturco, "How do you make a stent?" He replied, "Come into my workshop museum and give me thirty seconds and I will make one for you." We followed him downstairs to a room about twenty feet square. Along the entire back wall was a workbench filled with hand tools. Along the wall on the right was a variety of catheters hanging on hooks, while the wall on the left displayed his many degrees and honors.

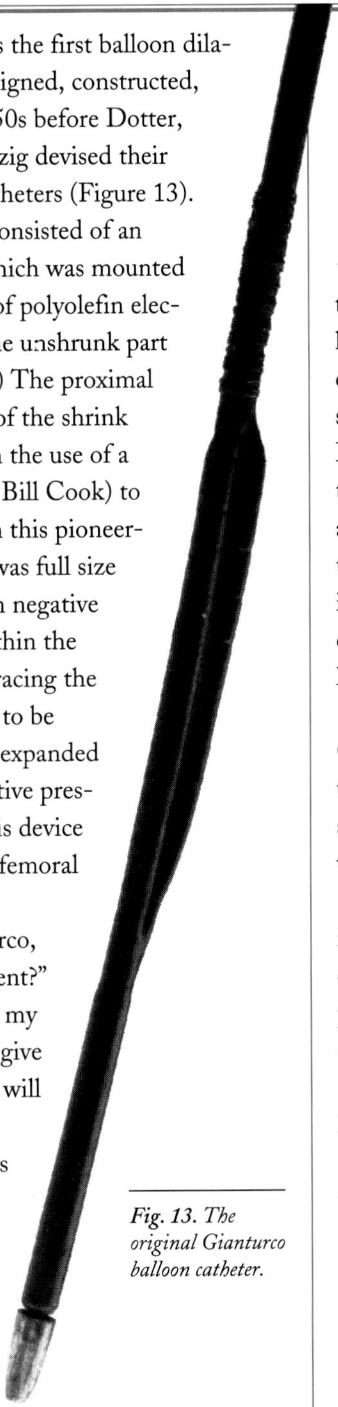

Fig. 13. The original Gianturco balloon catheter.

Gianturco removed a balloon catheter from a hook, took it to the workbench, and then picked up a spool of copper wire. With the left thumb holding the wire against the balloon, he completed a single turn. Then came a surprise because he repositioned his left thumb and made a second turn in the opposite direction. He continued winding each turn in opposite directions so that the coil had no complete turns. In fact, the coil consisted of U-shaped turns around the balloon. He stopped winding after the coil was about one inch long. Then he connected a syringe to the balloon port and said, "Watch." As the balloon inflated, the C-shaped coil expanded and its internal diameter could be determined by the amount of balloon inflation.

This remarkable device, the stainless steel Gianturco-Roubin Flex-Stent Coronary Stent, has undergone clinical trials with favorable results. The stent acts like an implanted scaffold, holding the vessel open and restoring blood flow to the tissue.

Gianturco also demonstrated one of his latest innovations—arterial plugs designed to close the hole of insertion when a large introducer sheath is used prior to angioplasty. A hole needed for insertion of a catheter as large as 9-French (which requires a 12-French sheath) can easily be plugged by a simple lump of material wrapped around a short pin.

In addition, he demonstrated a model of a septal defect occluder, which is designed to plug heart defects that might otherwise require open-heart surgery. The large plug is placed with two inner catheters and a sheath.

Cesare Gianturco remains one of the most innovative minds in medicine. His ideas and solutions to problems are truly unique, usually simple, and often not based on any of his preceding developments. He will never stop tinkering with new devices and coming up with new techniques. Undoubtedly, we have not seen the last of his work. Gianturco's "failure at retirement" continues to provide successes that benefit physicians and patients alike.

THE GIANTURCO-COOK PARTNERSHIP

Cesare Gianturco began working with Cook, Inc., in the late 1960s. A wide range of products has emerged over the years.
- Gianturco-Wallace Chemotherapy Pulser
- Occluding Spring Emboli (formerly Gianturco-Wallace-Anderson Arterial Embolization Set)
- Gianturco-Roehm Bird's Nest™ Vena Cava Filter
- Cook Z™ Stent (formerly Gianturco-Rösch Biliary Z-Stent)
- Gianturco-Roubin Flex-Stent™ Coronary Stent

The partnership between Gianturco and Cook, Inc. continues to this day, with several ideas in work.

A man likes
marvelous things;
so he invents them,
and is astonished.

Edgar Watson Howe

CHAPTER 10: Sidney Wallace

Applying Interventional Radiology to Cancer Treatment

Sidney Wallace has devoted his professional life to the diagnosis and treatment of cancer patients and has made important strides in applying interventional radiology to cancer treatment. He was among the first to recognize the potential of lymphangiography and subsequently had a tremendous influence on the development of intraarterial infusion, embolization, and chemoembolization as anticancer weapons.

Wallace began his career in medicine as a surgeon in the 1950s. In 1960, he began a residency in radiology and medicine at Jefferson Medical College of Thomas Jefferson University in Philadelphia, his hometown. While there, he pursued an interest in radiographic determination of the effects of certain cancerous tumors on lymph nodes. In 1961, Wallace and associates at Jefferson published a groundbreaking series of scientific papers on the diagnostic and therapeutic potential of lymphangiography that brought the importance of the procedure to the attention of radiologists.

As early as 1933, Hudack and McMaster used blue dye as a contrast agent to visualize the lymphatic system. In 1944, the surgeon Servelle dissected lymphatics, inserted a needle, and injected the agent Thorotrast. In 1952, Kinmouth and associates combined these procedures by introducing blue dye and performing a cut-down procedure, isolating the lymphatic vessel, inserting a needle, and injecting Thorotrast. (He eventually used a water-based contrast agent instead.) In 1958, Bruun and Engeset in Norway injected an oil-based contrast agent into a fistulous tract of the groin to make inguinal lymph nodes opaque.

Other forerunners of lymphangiography include Prokopek and Malek in Europe and Hreshchyshyn, Sheehan, and Holland at Roswell Park Hospital in Buffalo, New York, who injected Ethiodol, which is the ethyl ether of poppy seed oil. Wallace and his associates refined and improved the technique for visualizing the lymphatics and lymph nodes, making it more clinically applicable for diagnosing a wide range of diseases. Wallace points out that he built his methodology on the foundation of those who preceded him, just as Kinmouth had done before and others have done since.

Wallace's Technique

Wallace's technique for visualizing the lymphatics involved intradermal injection of dye followed by an incision to isolate the lymphatic. Wallace inserted a needle coupled to a polyethylene catheter and advanced it into the distended lymphatic channel. He then injected contrast agent and was able to get a clear view of the vessels within a few minutes, although the nodes are best visualized one day later. The primary criterion for a diagnosis of metastatic disease is a defect in a node not traversed by lymphatics. In their 1961 paper, Jackson, Wallace, and associates wrote about what they called the "rim sign," which is the residual functioning portion of the node that appears crescent in shape.

Wallace and his associates reported no complications in a 140-patient study in 1961, except for those due to improper injection technique. He judged lymphangiography to be an excellent method for following the changes in lymph nodes and providing a guide for the surgical treatment of tumors.

The technique was brought to a wider radiologic audience in 1965 when Wallace (with Dodd and Greening) published a chapter in *The Management of the Patient With Cancer*, a book edited by Nealon. The chapter documents the dynamics of lymph flow, the development of edema by blockage, the inverse relationship of the size to the number of lymph nodes at any given site, and the margins of a node that usually remain visible until there is total destruction by a tumor.

In the 1970s, Wallace and his associates at The University of Texas M.D. Anderson Hospital and Tumor Institute at Houston performed one of the first percutaneous lymph-node biopsies (Figure 1) and wrote the first paper on percutaneous biopsies of lymph nodes and other organs. They also performed paravascular biopsies of lymph nodes and ultimately published a number of articles on a wide range of lymph-node and tissue biopsies. Lymphangiography was the primary method of evaluating lymph nodes through the 1960s and 1970s, until the use of computed tomographic (CT) scanning caught on in the mid-1970s. The technique is now used less often, except in certain cancer hospitals, since new imaging devices are easier to use, results are simpler to interpret, and studies takes less time.

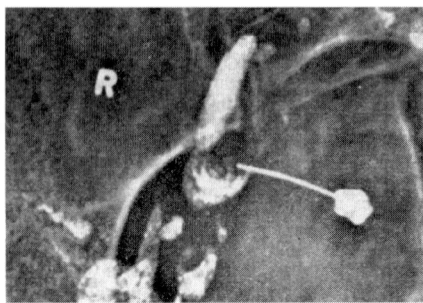

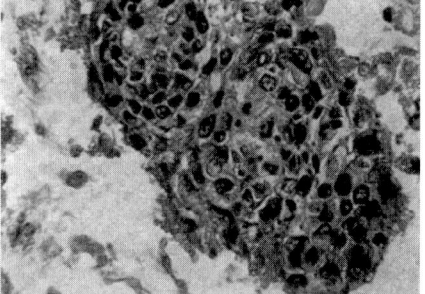

Fig. 1. Percutaneous aspiration biopsy of a lymph node (A) shows the biopsy in the area just above the crescent. (B) Squamous cell carcinoma revealed.

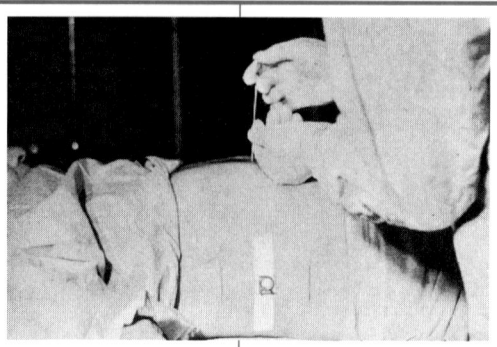

Fig. 2. In transhepatic cholangiography, a four-inch, plastic-sheathed needle was passed through the midaxillary line and bile aspirated. Wallace completed the first drainage by leaving the catheter in the common duct to drain the tract until surgery could be performed.

Drainage Firsts

From 1962 to 1963, Wallace (with Dodd and Greening) performed the first percutaneous transhepatic drainage of the biliary tract (Figure 2) and wrote about it in a chapter titled "The Radiologic Diagnosis of Cancer" for Nealon's book, *The Management of the Patient With Cancer*. Transhepatic cholangiography was first developed in Indochina prior to the 1960s. Dodd was one of the first to perform the technique in the United States. Wallace built on Dodd's methodology and completed the first drainage in the early 1960s, leaving the catheter in the common duct to drain the biliary tract. The patient was then treated by surgery.

In 1974, Wallace and his team at M.D. Anderson performed the first percutaneous abscess drainage of the liver and reported their results in the *American Journal of Roentgenology*. In 1953, the surgeon McFadzean had reported in the *British Journal of Surgery* that he and his colleagues accomplished liver drainage by cutting open the abdomen to locate the abscess and then inserting a needle through the skin to drain the abscess. Wallace and his associates were the first to accomplish the procedure without incisions, using radiography as their guide.

Infusion, Embolization, and Chemoembolization

Wallace has had a major influence on the therapeutic management of neoplasms with intraarterial infusion of chemotherapeutic agents, embolization, and chemoembolization. He has published numerous articles on all three methods.

Intraarterial infusion therapy—delivery of a chemotherapeutic agent directly into the artery that supplies the tumor—was first attempted in the 1950s. Wirtanen, a radiotherapist in Madison, Wisconsin, developed the technique by placing catheters for intraarterial infusion. Wallace and his colleagues refined the infusion techniques and managed to redistribute flow by putting coils into certain vessels and forcing a single vessel to be the primary supplier of the tumor. This accomplishment allowed a single catheter to be placed instead of multiple catheters and facilitated the delivery of chemotherapeutic agents to fewer vessels, preferably one.

Wallace and his M.D. Anderson team were instrumental in developing infusion techniques for a variety of tumors. Their most successful infusion therapy—and their biggest contribution to the field of chemotherapy—is used to treat osteosarcomas in teenagers. Wallace and his associates began that work in the late 1970s with a group of chemotherapists and surgeons, and their research continues today.

Embolization for Tumors

In 1952, Markowitz first proposed disrupting arterial blood supply to liver tumors to create tumor ischemia and arrest tumor growth. In 1970, the M.D. Anderson team attempted embolization of the hepatic artery to treat liver tumors. On their first attempt, they accidentally damaged the vessel. At first they were quite concerned that they may have injured the patient, but about a month later the patient returned for a follow-up visit and they found that the tumor had shrunk to about half its previous size. By injuring the vessel and starving the blood supply to the tumor, the researchers inadvertently decreased the size of the tumor—a most serendipitous discovery.

In describing the incident, Wallace said, "A lot of this is serendipity. You have to recognize the problem and change adversity to advantage. You have to try to use some of the problems that you create unknowingly for the benefit of the patient, as long as you don't harm the patient."

Wallace and his group used embolization for giant-cell bone tumors in another group of patients, a technique that is still used today. Small particles, usually Gelfoam and embolizing coils, were inserted into primary and collateral blood vessels. Many patients reported rapid and lasting pain relief. Tumors appeared to heal more rapidly, becoming more calcified and smaller after embolization.

Wallace first used embolization for bone tumors in 1975, when a sixteen-year-old female came to M.D. Anderson with a large tumor. She had previously tried a variety of therapies that proved to be ineffective. Wallace's team blocked the blood supply to the tumor; after seventeen years, the woman is still doing well.

Chemoembolization Discoveries

The goal of cancer chemotherapy is to deliver a high concentration of anticancer agent directly to the tumor and avoid providing high systemic concentrations of the agent. One method of reaching this goal is by using a catheter to deliver the agent directly into the artery that supplies the tumor. Although effective, the chemotherapeutic agent acts only as a "first-pass" effect when delivered intraarterially.

Chemoembolization is a method of prolonging contact time between the chemotherapeutic agent and the tumor tissue by combining intraarterial infusion of a chemotherapeutic agent and arterial embolization of the vascular supply to a neoplasm. This combination theoretically produces ischemia, decreases blood flow, and allows an

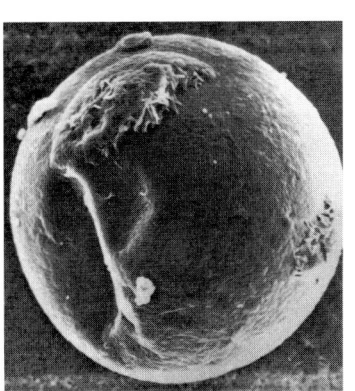
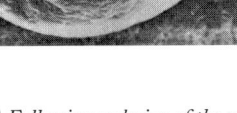

Fig. 3. (A) Following occlusion of the celiac artery, the collateral pathway was catheterized from the superior mesenteric artery through the inferior pancreatic duodenal artery to the gastroduodenal artery and then to the hepatic. (B) The internal mammary artery became a major supplier to the liver.

increase in contact time between the chemotherapeutic agent and the tumor. Ivalon (polyvinyl alcohol foam) particles, Gelfoam segments, and powder are often combined with cytotoxic agents. The procedure originated with the Japanese urologist Kato, who in 1981 used particles about 200 microns in size to demonstrate that chemoembolization with microcapsules containing chemotherapeutic agents was superior to local intraarterial injection of antitumor agents.

Chemoembolization has become an important method of treating patients with ocular melanoma, a tumor in the eye that spreads to the liver in 75% of patients. A patient can die in two months if hepatic metastasis occurs. Wallace and associates have extended that life span to as long as five years; the median survival time is eleven months. Wallace's technique is to embolize the hepatic artery with a combination of polyvinyl sponge particles and a suspension of cisplatin. Embolization of the hepatic artery is known to have an antineoplastic effect on primary and secondary hepatic neoplasms, while cisplatin has shown some promise against melanoma when given intraarterially.

Wallace believed that the effect of the polyvinyl sponge and the activity of the cisplatin would be synergistic, with the sponge slowing down blood flow and prolonging the time the neoplastic cells are exposed to higher concentrations of cisplatin. After one or two treatments, patients experience a dramatic regression of the hepatic metastases with a longer duration of remission. Certain tumors, such as metastatic neuroendocrine tumors, are still primarily treated by embolization and now by chemoembolization.

Microencapsulation

Wallace was fascinated by the potential of microencapsulation, the process of creating small particles and filling them with different materials, mostly pharmaceutical compounds. The microcapsules can be made in almost any size, usually from 1 to 1,000 microns, but the standard size is either 1 micron or 100 microns (the 100-micron size is used for chemoembolization, Figure 4). The National Cash Register Company holds most of the patents on microencapsulation technology, and many of their patents are for products used in everyday life. For example, when you sign a carbonless paper, the weight of the pen fractures tiny particles (microcapsules) filled with "ink" that make the imprint.

Wallace started making microcapsules in 1975 after meeting Benjamin Mosier at a cocktail party and asking him about his occupation. As fate would have it, Mosier was a physical chemist who made particles containing barium for use by oil companies. The particles were dropped to the bottom of old oil wells to float up previously unpumped oil. Wallace was not working on anything related to microencapsulation yet, but something clicked in his mind when Mosier was describing his line of work. He suggested to Mosier that the two combine forces to make particles for use in the arteries and veins.

Wallace and Mosier worked many years together. Mosier never told Wallace exactly what he was doing—he just made the material and brought it in for testing. On some days, every test animal died because the basic method they used was a solvent evaporation technique. If Mosier didn't wash all the toxic solvents off, the toxicity would kill the animals. The two men made a variety of materials, including contrast agents used in radiology and chemotherapeutic agents.

In 1985, Mosier obtained a patent on his method of placing anticancer agents into microcapsules that could lodge in a tumor because the capsules were larger than red blood cells. In studies with heparinized dog blood, Mosier found that the rate of drug release did not depend on either capsule size or capsule

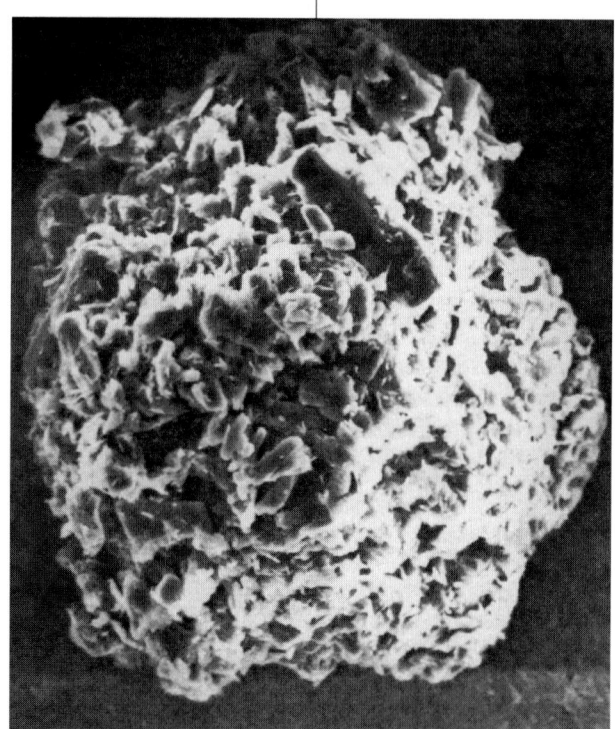

Fig. 4. Microencapsulated particles may carry a wide variety of agents.

content. However, the total amount of drug released was dependent on both capsule size and content. Wallace and Mosier's microcapsules could be tailor-made for the desired release rate and the total amount of drug to be delivered.

Wallace found many uses for microencapsulation. One involved the blockage of vessels that supply blood to tumors. Since the maximum tumor vessel size is about 100 microns, a particle was created a little larger than 100 microns to block the vessel feeding blood to the tumor. Another use involved the lymphatics. The average pore size of the lymphatics in the peritoneal cavity is about 500 microns. Wallace created a microcapsule larger than 500 microns to keep the capsule inside the cavity. Wallace also created microcapsules smaller than 5 microns in size, smaller than the size of capillaries, so that they could be injected into a vein and travel through the lungs.

Work with David Yang

When Wallace brought in chemist David Yang in the late 1980s to add consistency to the making of microcapsules, Mosier parted company with Wallace. Wallace and Yang developed a consistent, nontoxic method of encapsulating a variety of contrast materials, including Ethiodol, Telepaque, and ionic and nonionic water-based contrast media.

Wallace and Yang also encapsulated contrast materials that had only been used orally because they were too toxic. The body tolerates intravenous injections of encapsulated contrast material because the material is protected by the capsule. In essence, Wallace and Yang created a sustained-release drug delivery system.

The two scientists have used Telepaque, a common contrast material that is usually taken orally to visualize the gallbladder, because it is easily administered intravenously when encapsulated. Telepaque is extremely dense, and most of it goes to the liver, where it is disposed of either through the urine or feces. Its release is sustained from the time of initial injection, and the speed of release depends on the capsular material, the ratio of the amount of contrast agent to the size of the capsule, and the thickness of the capsular wall. The speed of release can be changed by altering these parameters or the size of the particle.

Wallace and Yang have tested four different contrast agents and are working to create a functional encapsulated nonionic contrast material.

They have put almost every type of chemotherapeutic agent in capsules for chemoembolization of large particles and for intravenous or intraarterial delivery of small particles. More recently, they have added an extra coat to the particles to help target specific sites. They have applied for a patent on one of the coating materials used in microencapsulation by solvent evaporation. If particles less than 5 microns in size (usually about 3 microns or less) are coated with polylactic acid and injected, the particles will usually be picked up by Kupffer cells, the protective macrophage cells in the liver that take abnormal materials out of the blood circulation. If the particles are given a coat of phenylalanine on top of the polylactic acid, the particles will be targeted to hepatocytes and not to Kupffer cells.

Tamoxifen and Estrogen-Receptor Sites

Wallace and Yang have wrapped particles in estrone, an estrogen-like material, to increase their intake in the uterus and ovaries, which are estrogen-receptor sites. They have also applied for a patent on analogs of tamoxifen. Tamoxifen is a drug that competes with estrogen for estrogen-receptor sites in the body.

Tamoxifen is commonly used in the treatment of breast cancer in postmenopausal women. About 60% of breast cancers have estrogen-receptor positivity because they involve estrogen-receptor sites. Tamoxifen binds to those sites as it competes with estrogen. It is consequently able to get into the cell cytoplasm and kill the cell. About half of the women with estrogen-receptor positivity can be treated successfully with tamoxifen.

Altering Tamoxifen

Wallace and Yang have used tamoxifen because of its extensive application to a large percentage of postmenopausal breast-cancer patients; however, they have altered the drug by adding a halogen and sulfhydryls. Tamoxifen's makeup is easily changed by halogenation. Wallace and Yang made the compound so simple that it takes just two steps to change from its initial form to halogenated tamoxifen.

Tamoxifen can easily be changed to a halogenated or radioactive halogenated form. Both forms have as much as 150 times the binding power to estrogen-receptor sites and twenty-three times the killing power as tamoxifen alone. Care must be taken that the toxicity is also not twenty-three times greater. Each halogen has two forms: a sys and a trans form. The sys form has greater killing power, while the trans form has greater binding power.

Some of the first experiments Wallace and Yang undertook included adding fluorine-18 (an isotope of fluorine) to fluorinated tamoxifen instead of adding fluorine; they used the experiment for a PET (positron emission tomography) study, a procedure they feel has tremendous potential. With the use of fluorotamoxifen, a PET camera identified the uterus and ovaries, something that had not been possible in prior PET studies. The uterus and ovaries can be seen by a PET camera because the fluorotamoxifen attaches to the estrogen-receptor sites in the uterus and ovaries.

Since tamoxifen has binding power and killing power in an estrogen-receptor site, Wallace and Yang plan to put halogenated tamoxifen on the surface of microcapsules to bring the particles to the site and then release whatever chemotherapeutic drug is inside.

Teaming Up with Cesare Gianturco

In 1968, when the great interventionalist Cesare Gianturco retired from the Carle Clinic in Urbana, Illinois, at age sixty-two, he accepted an invitation to join Wallace and the M.D. Anderson team for six months out of each year. At first Gianturco wanted to do lymphangiography, especially since Wallace was one of the pioneers in the procedure. However, lymphangiography required putting a needle into a very tiny vessel. As Wallace points out, the procedure is akin to "giving an enema to a flea." He remembers how Gianturco would wear three pairs of glasses in order to see the lymphatic vessel.

Gianturco helped Wallace and Dodd create a laboratory in the department of diagnostic radiology that emphasized interventional radiology. Their first project involved the use of heparin for angiography, following up on the work Gianturco had done with Stegarta in Illinois. The M.D. Anderson group repeated Gianturco's experiments in its laboratory and then performed the work on patients and published a paper in 1970 on systemic heparinization for angiography. They

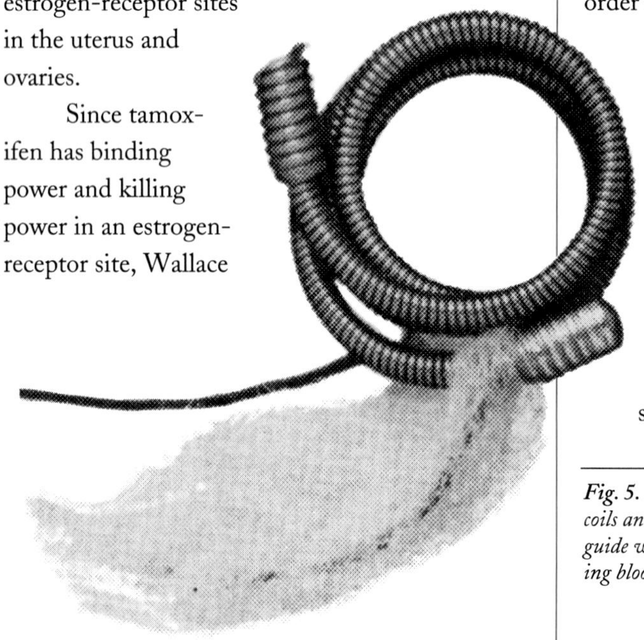

Fig. 5. Wallace and Gianturco teamed up to develop a variety of coils and stents. This minicoil was made of stainless steel. When the guide wire was removed, the coil wound itself up, effectively blocking blood flow in the penetrated vessel.

also produced an exhibit for a meeting of the Radiological Society of North America about the surface characteristics of catheters, wires, and guides to show that it is important to use heparin to protect the patient's body against clots.

Besides their work on heparinization, Wallace and Gianturco have done quite a bit of work on coils (Figure 5) and stents (Figures 6 and 7), much of which is discussed in greater detail in the chapter on Gianturco. They also did some preliminary work together on the Bird's Nest filter. In 1973, Wallace and Gianturco first worked on wool coils and modified the coils two years later to make them more applicable to a variety of clinical situations. They discussed the coils' use in blocking a tumor in the liver and then used them in a variety of different ways to change blood supply to organs— "redistributing the blood supply," as they called it. They were the first to use coils to close fistulas in a variety of different vascular circumstances. Though the woolly-tail embolizing coils were originally made with wool, the product is now manufactured with Dacron.

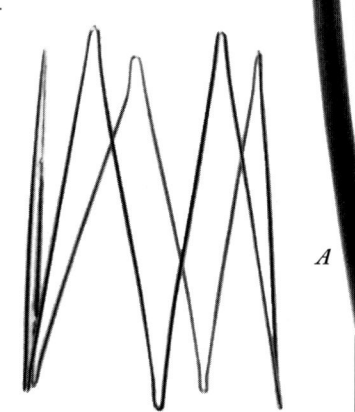

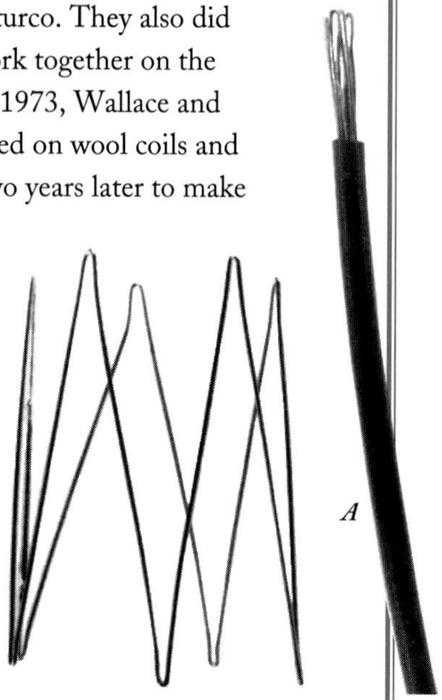

Fig. 6. Wallace and Gianturco experimented with stainless steel stents. (A) Shows the collapsed stent beginning to exit the Teflon sheath. (B) Demonstrates the expansion after the stent is pushed completely from the sheath.

Wallace remembers that the wool for the early coils came out of Mrs. Gianturco's sewing basket. Wallace laughs when recounting that she "lost" a number of items from that basket to her husband's ability to make just about anything with some wire and a pair of pliers.

Wallace was impressed with the simplicity of many of the devices Gianturco made at M.D. Anderson. One was a device for delivering barium during an enema that enabled the physician to stand at a distance instead of standing by the patient's side. Reasoning that since fluoroscopy can be done from a distance, Gianturco devised a simple string and pulley system in which the string could be pulled from behind a shield. The delivery tube would kink when the string was pulled. When he wanted to release the tube, Gianturco would just pull it down, and the tube would open again. One day a visitor from Sweden proudly told Wallace of a fancy gadget he had made to give barium enemas remotely. Wallace showed him Gianturco's device, which was much simpler and more efficient.

After the coils were developed, Wallace told Gianturco, "Cesare, now is our chance. We have to go on to opening up the vessels." That was the preliminary inspiration for Gianturco's work on stents. About five years later, in 1985, Gianturco came back with his design for the zigzag stent, and the M.D. Anderson team has been working on stents ever since.

Although Rösch was the first to tie two stents together, the original design was by Gianturco, who used a single stent, then two separate stents, and then two stents tied together with a strut. He then added barbs to keep the stent in place. Wallace and Gianturco have been working on stents for the tracheobronchial tree, venous system, and biliary tract. All of the basic work has been done in the M.D. Anderson laboratory, including the work on Gianturco's biliary stent.

Wallace admits that working with Gianturco has been quite an educational experience and that Gianturco is the genius behind many of their developments. Gianturco has brought decades of innovative thought and knowledge to the M.D. Anderson group. Wallace says that on more than one occasion, he has gotten an idea while Gianturco was with him in the lab, causing Gianturco to respond, "Forget it. I tried it forty years ago and it was no damn good." Wallace would reply with something on the order of, "Now for the first time you will get it right." The give and take between the two has resulted in some impressive contributions to the field of intervention.

About Wallace

Sidney Wallace literally grew up in a meat market; his father was a kosher butcher. Sidney started developing his surgical technique as a child by boning meat, and he admits to having plucked millions of chickens with great aplomb. Having learned basic surgical technique from countless slabs of beef, veal, and lamb, he felt it was a natural transition to go from the meat market into surgery.

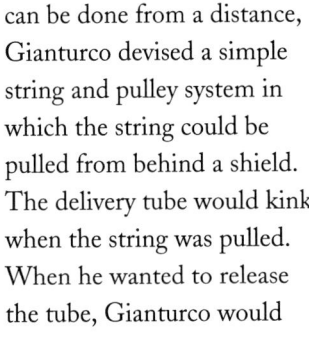
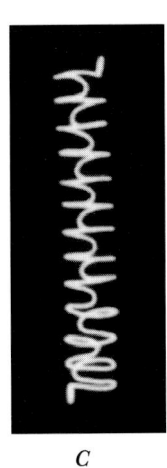

Fig. 7. Wallace tried a balloon-expanded stainless steel stent in the 1980s. (A) reveals the angioplasty balloon-stent in the collapsed state. (B) shows the stent after inflation. (C) The expanded stent remains after the angioplasty balloon is withdrawn.

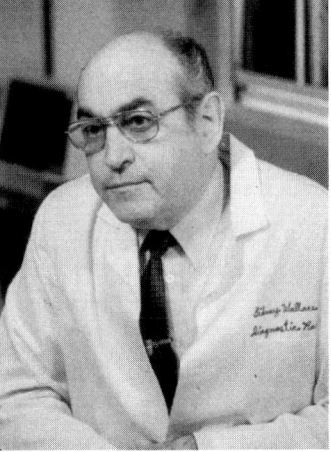

Fig. 8. Sidney Wallace

FOCUSING ON THE PATIENT

Although much of his early work was with devices and his present focus is on chemicals and pharmaceuticals, Wallace's primary concern has always been patients and the effects of disease on them. A great deal of his research has been on the management of tumors, which holds a special interest for him. "The number of people working in the management of the cancer patient is really very small," Wallace says. "It takes time, it takes extra effort, it takes an environment like M.D. Anderson, it takes a multidisciplinary teamwork approach....Our whole bit is the treatment of cancer patients."

THE WALLACE-COOK PARTNERSHIP

Sidney Wallace and Cook Incorporated have enjoyed a productive partnership for over two decades. Among the innovations resulting from this teamwork are the following:
- Gianturco-Wallace Chemotherapy Pulser
- Occluding Spring Emboli (formerly the Gianturco-Wallace-Anderson Arterial Embolization Set)

The pas de deux of Wallace and Cook Incorporated that has been so beneficial to interventional radiology continues. Significant projects are in progress as this book goes to press.

Wallace received a B.A. degree from Temple University in 1949 and his M.D. degree from that same hometown institution in 1954. He followed an internship at Philadelphia General Hospital with a one-year surgical residency there, where he set a record in obstetrics by delivering seventeen babies in one night. After that, he spent one year as a surgeon in Philadelphia before entering the U.S. Army.

Wallace was in the Army at the end of the Korean War. He went to Japan to perform surgery from 1956 to 1958. At the time, the Army sent single doctors stationed in Japan to Korea. Wallace went with an obstetrician, a gynecologist, and a pediatrician. The group mostly performed pediatrics and treated many contagious diseases. Many of the soldiers caught childhood diseases while they were away from home for the first time. Wallace was stationed on the 38th Parallel for three months, working as a surgeon in a MASH unit. Since the war was over, there were few casualties to contend with. Much of their emergency duty involved taking care of soldiers who accidentally shot themselves or each other.

When he got out of the Army, Wallace spent six months as a surgical instructor at Lower Bucks County Hospital outside Philadelphia, when he decided to enter the field of radiology. He says, "I decided to see the light . . . or darkness . . . however you want to look at it." He started his residency in radiology at Jefferson Medical College of Thomas Jefferson University, followed by a one-year fellowship in radiology with Boijsen in Lund, Sweden, from 1963 to 1964.

Back to "Meat"

While a resident at Jefferson, Wallace received a visit from his mother. When she first saw him decked out in red goggles, a long apron, and big gloves, she exclaimed, "Oh my God, you're back in the meat market!"

When he returned from Sweden, Wallace was appointed to the staff of Jefferson Medical College as an instructor and then assistant professor. In 1966, he joined the staff of The University of Texas M.D. Anderson Hospital and Tumor Institute at Houston (since renamed The University of Texas M.D. Anderson Cancer Center), first as an associate professor, then gaining the rank of professor in 1969.

At present, Sidney Wallace is professor of radiology and chairman of the department of diagnostic imaging at M.D. Anderson. He also holds the John S. Dunn, Sr., Chair. The laboratory in which he works was established by a gift from the late John S. Dunn and is supported by the Dunn Foundation for Immunologic Sciences. The Dunn Laboratory provides support for research on new devices and techniques for interventional radiology. Cook Incorporated is a supporter of the Dunn Laboratory and its research and therapeutic activities. Wallace's ability to develop new methods and uses for selective placement of microcapsules, stents, and other materials into various areas of the vascular system has been honed to perfection by his continuing research activity in the Dunn Laboratory.

Wallace has major administrative, teaching, and clinical responsibilities as head of diagnostic radiology at M.D. Anderson. There are thirty staff radiologists and an equal number of residents and fellows within the department. It is not unusual for him to conduct early morning discussion and teaching sessions on the day's upcoming cases or the patients examined the previous day.

Over the years, his pioneering diagnostic and therapeutic uses of interventional radiology have earned him the recognition and respect of his colleagues. He has received numerous honors for his work, including the French Antoine Beclerc award and awards from the American Roentgen Ray Society, the American Medical Association, the Radiological Society of North America, and other societies. He has accepted many lectureships and has served as a reviewer and on the advisory editorial boards for leading professional journals in his field.

In 1958, Sidney Wallace met Marsha Joan Baker and married her the following year in Atlantic City, New Jersey. They are the parents of two sons (one a music composer and the other a radiologist and sculptor) and one daughter (a motion picture costume designer).

Radiology and Art

Work is Wallace's hobby. However, he finds time for such artistic activities as sculpting, painting, and music. He has drawn cartoons since his childhood and says, "If I painted a sign that said, 'Hamburger, 25 cents a pound,' my father thought that was great. If I did cartoons, he thought I was wasting my time."

Wallace places much importance in his faith. He serves as a synagogue cantor and assists his wife in helping Jewish refugees immigrate to the United States.

Wallace points out that the number of people working on the management of cancer patients is rather small. He recognizes it takes time, extra effort, and an environment like M.D. Anderson, where a multidisciplinary team approach has many people working together for the benefit of the patient.

Wallace regards his biggest contribution to interventional radiology to be his work in intraarterial infusion, embolization, and chemoembolization for treating cancer patients. He emphasizes that the treatment of cancer patients is the sole purpose of his work.

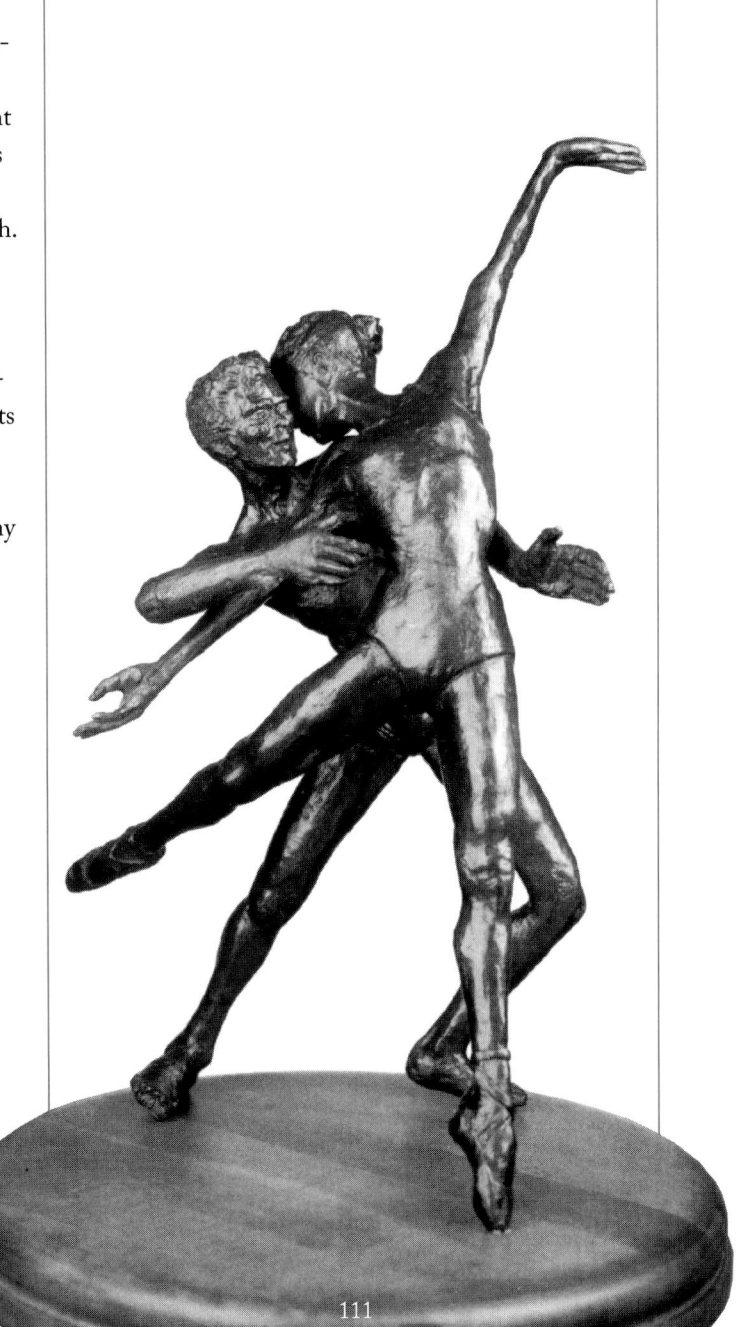

Fig. 9. Wallace created this bronze sculpture in the early 1980s. It stands about 18 inches tall.

Now, boys, we have got her done. Let's start her up and see why she doesn't work.

John Fritz

CHAPTER 11: Constantin Cope

Pioneering Contributions To Diagnostic Techniques

Constantin Cope has combined his creative mind and fascination with gadgets to make enormous contributions to the fields of angiography and interventional radiology. Although trained as an internist, Cope chose to specialize in angiography to help make more accurate diagnoses with less invasive methods and devices. During his residency training in 1955, for example, he noted that it was impossible for physicians to distinguish pancreatic cancer from hepatitis in jaundiced patients. If the patient responded to treatment, the diagnosis was hepatitis. Conversely, if a patient's condition worsened, the diagnosis was cancer. Cope believed there was a better way.

Large Bore Catheters

When he published his first scientific paper on a new method of introducing large bore catheters, Cope could not have realized the impact he was to have on the yet-to-be-named field of interventional radiology. The paper, published in the *New England Journal of Medicine* in 1958, informed the medical community that a modified large bore catheter was a valuable tool for intravenous therapy, angiography, thoracentesis, abdominal paracentesis, and drainage. At the time his paper was published, physicians considered large bore catheters difficult to introduce, and consequently they rarely used them.

To solve the problems inherent to the introduction of large bore catheters, Cope developed a catheter-needle. He passed a length of tubing over a 14-gauge needle 25 cm long and drew the distal portion down so that the inner diameter of the catheter was the same as the diameter of the needle, as shown in Figure 1. Cope then cut the catheter to expose from 2 to 3 mm of the beveled tip of the needle. He inserted the catheter-needle through a nick in the patient's skin, and when the catheter-needle was in the

Fig. 1. Cope's method of drawing tubing so that it fits snugly over a 14-gauge needle (A, B). Cope inserted the needle through a nick in the patient's skin and advanced it to the desired vessel or viscus.

desired vessel or viscus, he withdrew the needle, advanced the catheter, and affixed the catheter to a cannula.

The ability of Cope's catheter-needle to enlarge the opening in a patient's skin was a significant development. Cope pioneered the use of tapered catheter tips to gradually enlarge the puncture hole for the catheter and allow a large bore catheter to be introduced easily.

A New Biopsy Device

In 1958, Cope's interest in angiography led him to undertake a year of training in pulmonary diseases at the VA Hospital in East Orange, New Jersey, so he could practice angiographic techniques. While he was a resident on the tuberculosis service there, Cope created a biopsy device designed to help improve the methods used to obtain specimens of pleura. The device had three parts: a needle (Figure 2A), a cannula with a sharpened end (Figure 2B), and a curet with a slot on one end that was hooked (Figure 2C).

The technique Cope devised to obtain a pleural specimen was to nick the patient's skin with a scalpel first, then introduce the cannula and needle until pleural fluid was drawn by syringe aspiration. He then withdrew the needle slightly until gentle syringe suction failed to provide any more fluid, which showed that the cannula was just outside the pleura. He removed the inner needle and introduced the curet, which was attached to a 2-ml syringe, to the hilt or until fluid was obtained. To obtain a good bite, he pushed the instrument laterally in the direction of the hooked slot in the curet. This maneuver fed pleural and subpleural tissue into the side opening of the curet. He then pulled the curet out gently until it caught the parietal pleura with its hook. Cope advanced the cannula with his other hand using a rotating motion until the cannula cut a small plug of tissue; then he could withdraw the assembly easily. With his biopsy device, Cope could obtain a specimen approximately 2 mm by 3 mm, containing pleural and subpleural tissue.

Commenting on the efficacy of his needle-biopsy instrument, Cope said, "The instrument has been used on ten patients without any morbidity. The instrument is well adapted for use in thoracentesis because of its blunt end. Thus it has become my custom to tap all pleural effusions with the needle and, just before withdrawal, cut a small plug of tissue, thereby accomplishing both duties in one operation."

The Cope hooked biopsy needle, as it became known after its introduction in 1958, was made available by Becton-Dickinson. It was subsequently used to obtain biopsy specimens from other tissues. In 1963, Cope and Bernhardt reported that it could be used to sample specimens from the pericardium, peritoneum, and synovium as well as from the pleura.

In reflecting on the success of the biopsy device, Cope said, "The hooked-needle biopsy was my first significant contribution, coming in 1958 when I was thirty years old. I was thrilled that my little trick was being accepted by other physicians without my trying to sell it in any way."

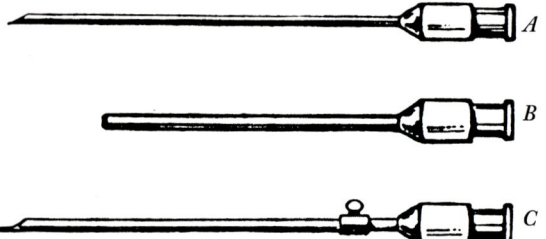

Fig. 2. Cope's needle-biopsy device consists of a needle (A), a cannula with a sharpened circular end (B), and a hooked curet (C).

The Transseptal Technique

In the 1950s, catheterization of the pulmonary artery to obtain pulmonary capillary wedge pressure was the only method available to determine pressure in the left atrium. Since this measurement was often inaccurate, scientists devised new technologies that allowed direct pressure measurement of the left heart.

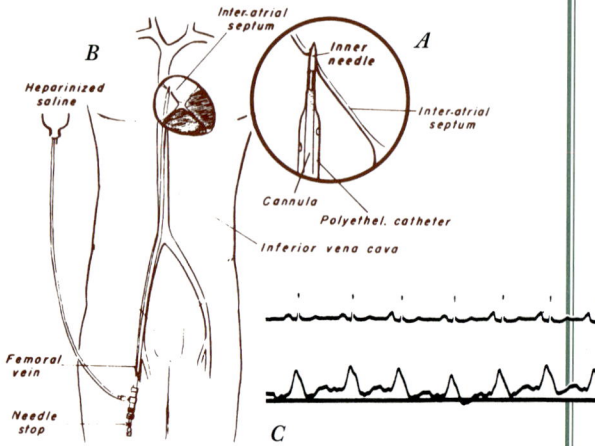

Fig. 3. These drawings illustrate Cope's transseptal technique. The drawing in the circle (A) shows the tip of a 70-cm long needle protruding from a tapered polyethylene catheter. Sketch (B) shows the route taken by the catheter-clad needle up the femoral vein. (C) illustrates the ECG and left atrial pressure recorded with the catheter tip in the left atrium.

Prior to Cope's development of the transseptal technique to measure left atrial or ventricular pressure, a number of somewhat dangerous methods were used. One involved introducing a long needle into the heart through the trachea. Another was a translumbar technique that involved introducing the needle into the heart through the patient's back. It seemed obvious to Cope that a safer method had to be found.

In 1959, he developed an alternative approach in which he accessed the left atrium by passing a 70-cm long, 17-gauge needle up the inferior vena cava, as shown in Figure 3. Cope covered the needle with polyethylene tubing drawn to fit snugly at the tip of the beveled needle, which protruded 2 to 3 mm. He also fitted the needle with a stylet and passed a catheter-needle up the inferior vena cava (Figure 3A) under fluoroscopic observation. When the tip came into contact with the atrial septum (Figure 3B), Cope advanced the stylet to enter the left atrium and record pressure. Figure 3C shows one of Cope's left atrial pressure records obtained from a patient with early mitral stenosis.

Recording left atrial pressure aided in the diagnosis of mitral stenosis. In addition, according to Cope, "The catheter can be used for sampling pressures within the left atrium and possibly within the left ventricle if a suitable polyethylene tube is passed through the catheter and allowed to float past the mitral valve." Cope's transseptal catheter-needle was commercially produced by Becton-Dickinson (Figure 4). His transseptal technique was later adapted to measure hemodynamics within the left heart. However, a retrograde catheter technique through the aortic valve became popular for valve transplants because many physicians had

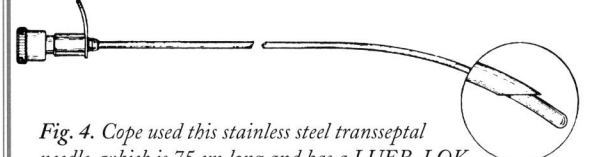

Fig. 4. Cope used this stainless steel transseptal needle, which is 75 cm long and has a LUER-LOK hub and a curve indicator. The inner obturator is a stainless steel 0.25-inch O.D. wire. The proximal end includes a male LUER-LOK hub that locks into the hub of the needle and prevents retraction of the obturator.

problems handling the transseptal technique, probably due to the fact that they were schooled in the transcatheter technique through the aorta.

As a result, the left atrial and transseptal technique fell into relative disuse, but during the middle to late 1980s, Cope's transseptal technique made a comeback when it was used to introduce dilation balloon catheters into the left atrium and left ventricle for the treatment of mitral and aortic stenoses.

Improvements in Catheterization

Recognizing the need to bend straight catheters, Cope created a small catheter guide in 1961. Using the same principle as that of a large Rappaport guide, Cope developed an instrument that could bend a catheter by applying tension to an inside wire. The guide consisted of three parts: (1) a 45- to 65-cm length of 20-gauge tubing soldered to a needle hub ground down to one-fifth of its diameter for a length of 3 to 5 cm; (2) a length of 20-gauge tubing containing slots cut to form ringlets; and (3) a length of 32-gauge stainless steel suture wire.

Cope placed the tube with the ringlets over the tip of the long tubing and soldered it into position. He attached the steel wire to the rounded flexible end and passed it up the long tubing to exit the needle hub. Figure 5 illustrates the three components and the curling effect produced by pulling on the ring (Figure 5B), which was connected to the stainless steel suture joined to the rounded tip (Figure 5A).

Cope used his steering device to guide catheters into arterial and venous ostia in dogs weighing from thirty to forty pounds. He recommended that the diameter of the polyethylene catheter always be reduced at the tip to contain the steering device.

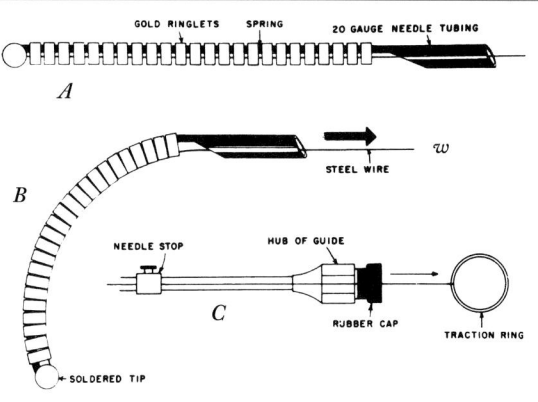

Fig. 5. This illustrates Cope's catheter guiding device. (A) shows the ringlets, which were made by slotting needle tubing affixed to a long needle (right). A stainless steel suture wire (w), affixed to the spherical end, exits the needle hub. (B) shows the curl produced by applying tension to the wire. (C) illustrates a needle stop to aid in placement.

The Cournand Needle Modification

The Cournand needle had gained preeminence as a device for drawing arterial blood samples. It employed a short length of needle tubing that protruded from the hub. However, once the physician obtained a blood sample, the stylet was difficult to insert because the field became obscured by blood.

In 1962, Cope solved the problem of reintroducing the stylet by grinding the protruding tubing and flattening it slightly to create a shelf, as shown in Figure 6. Even when the shelf was obscured by blood, the stylet could be guided into the needle by tactile sensation.

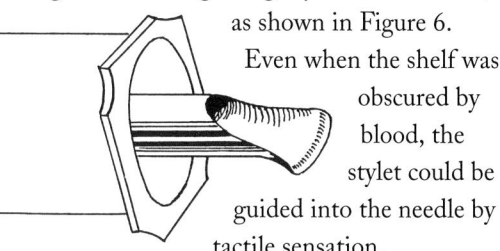

Fig. 6. Cope's modification of the Cournand needle permits easy reintroduction of the stylet after a blood sample has been aspirated into a syringe.

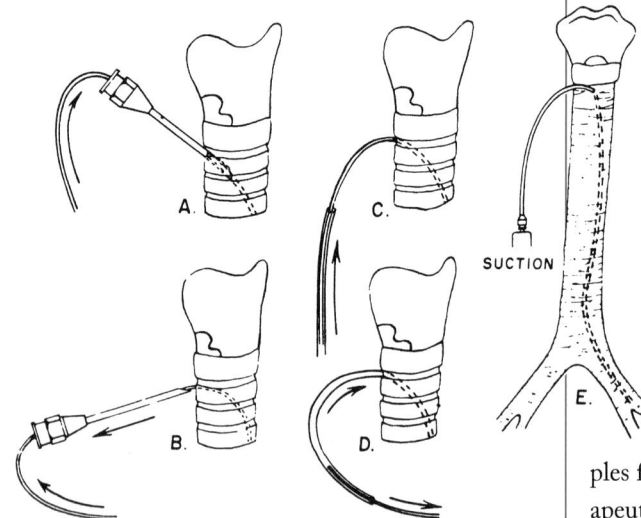

Fig. 7. Cope used the Seldinger technique to catheterize the trachebronchial tree in the sequence shown above.

Transtracheal Catheterization

In 1966, Cope became the first to use the Seldinger technique to access the tracheobronchial tree. Identifying several disadvantages of the nasal and oral approaches, he pointed out that the transtracheal approach eliminated most of these difficulties and was better tolerated by elderly patients.

Figure 7 illustrates the steps involved in transtracheal catheterization. Cope's approach was to place the patient on a radiographic table after the patient was sedated and given atropine. He inserted a 21-gauge needle into the trachea and injected lidocaine. Cope then exchanged that needle for a curved 17-gauge Teflon needle that consisted of a 4-inch, curved, 18-gauge needle with a solid bayonet point surrounded by a tightly fitting Teflon sleeve. Once the needle was properly positioned, he removed it, leaving the flexible Teflon catheter in place. Cope then inserted a guide wire into the lower trachea and removed the catheter.

Then he threaded a 20-cm nonradiopaque thin-walled Teflon catheter with a slightly tapered tip over the guide wire and advanced it into the lower trachea. He pulled the guide wire out and filled the catheter with contrast medium so that it could be visualized and directed fluoroscopically to the desired site.

Cope reported using the transtracheal catheter technique for more than one hundred patients with only one complication. Among the many advantages of the method was an ability to obtain uncontaminated fluid samples from the catheterized site and deliver chemotherapeutic agents to the site.

At least in part, Cope's success can be attributed to his strong sense of determination. He was so anxious to work with Seldinger wires that he couldn't wait the three months it took for them to be shipped from Sweden. Cope fashioned his own guide wires out of guitar strings until the Seldinger wires arrived.

Advances in Selective Aortography

In 1967, Cope addressed the complications resulting from extravasation of contrast agent through the walls of the external iliac arteries. To solve these problems, he developed a cannula that ensured forward flow of the contrast agent, which he accomplished by passing a fine wire with a 2-cm long, 18-gauge

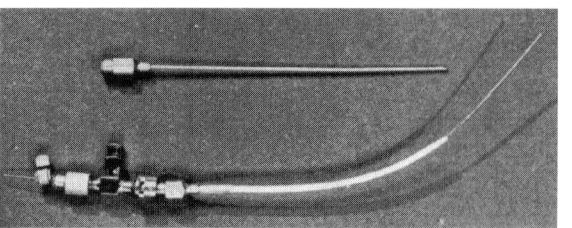

springy tip through the cannula in the vessel, thereby aligning the tip of the cannula with the vessel. Figure 8 illustrates successful and unsuccessful aortograms using this technique, as well as the Teflon cannula assembly.

Steerable Catheter System

In an effort to eliminate the need for an inventory of curved selective aortography catheters, Cope developed a steerable catheter system in 1969. This catheter assembly consisted of a thin-walled, 6-French polyethylene catheter whose distal portion was preformed in a C shape that was 3 cm in diameter (Figure 9). Inside this catheter were two wires—a curved 0.36-mm steerable wire and a straight wire, which was called the anti-flipper.

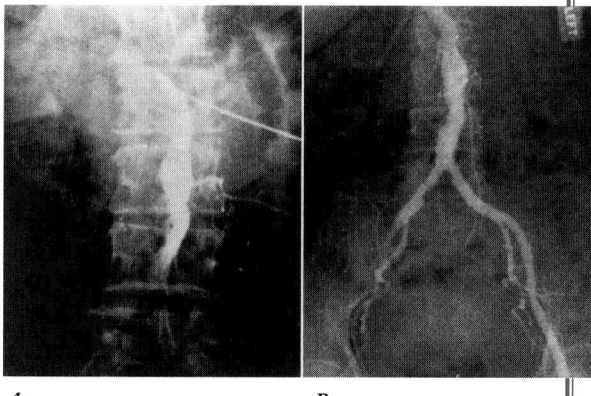

Fig. 8. Above (A): Extravasation of a 3-ml test dose of contrast medium during an unsuccessful translumbar aortogram. Above (B): Two days later, a retrograde power femoral aortogram in the same patient shows good filling of the lower and iliac arteries. Left: Cope developed this assembly to ensure forward flow of the contrast medium. (A) is the needle used to introduce the Teflon cannula into the artery. A special artery needle could also be used. (B) shows the Teflon cannula, adapter, and spring-tipped device, assembled for use. Note that the flexible tip protrudes beyond the cannula. The coil aligns the cannula in the vessel for forward flow of the contrast agent.

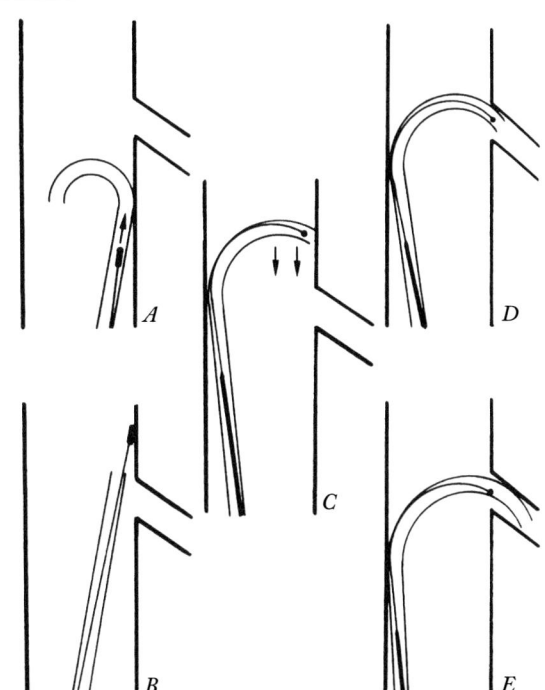

Fig. 9. Cope's torque-control catheter consists of a thin-walled 6-French polyethylene catheter with a C-shaped tip containing a wire in a similar C shape. The guide wire straightens the C tip (A, B, C), allowing placement of the tip in the desired vessel (D, E).

Cope inserted the anti-flipper to straighten the curved catheter and allow an aortogram to be made; he introduced the torque control wire for selective study. This system required only one catheter for both aortographic and selective studies.

Over a four-year period, Cope reported successful placement of his steerable catheter to visualize branches of the abdominal aorta. Only a few seconds were required to catheterize the desired site. By reducing the time required for selective catheterization, Cope effectively reduced vessel wall trauma and the need for large amounts of contrast agent.

Drainage Improvements

It disturbed Cope that a Foley or Malecot nephrostomy drainage catheter often became dislodged and was difficult to reinsert. So in 1980 he developed a simple drainage catheter to alleviate these problems. Starting with an 11-French perforated polyvinyl catheter, he passed a plastic suture inside and brought it out through the proximal perforation, about 7 to 11 cm from the catheter tip. The end of the suture was affixed to the tip of the catheter. Therefore, the suture stayed inside the catheter until it emerged from the proximal hole, then ran alongside to the catheter where it was affixed to the tip, as shown in Figure 10. The device became known as the crossed-limb loop (CLL) catheter.

Cope introduced the CLL catheter through a percutaneous nephrostomy tract that had been dilated. He then advanced the CLL catheter in the renal pelvis (Figure 10A), after which he simultaneously pulled gently on the suture and rotated the catheter clockwise along its long axis. Fluoroscopic visualization revealed that the catheter tip formed a loop in the renal pelvis (Figure 10B). Cope pulled the suture until the catheter tip was against the proximal hole of the catheter (Figure 10C). Since the end portion of the catheter was virtually a closed loop, the catheter had excellent self-retention. Finally, Cope secured the external end of the suture to the hub of the catheter, as shown in Figure 10C. No retaining skin sutures were required to keep the CLL drainage catheter in place. To remove the catheter, Cope severed the tethering suture, causing the loop to uncoil; then he gently withdrew the catheter.

In 1980, Cope reported using this 11-French drainage catheter in twenty-five patients without accidental withdrawal, except for one time when the

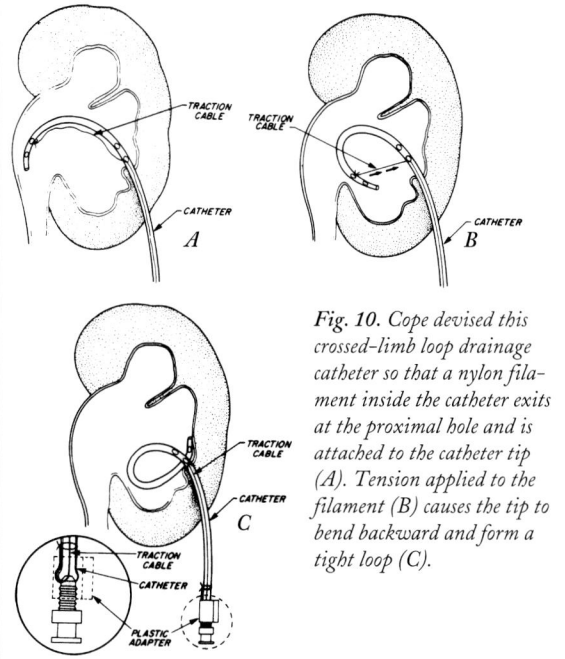

Fig. 10. Cope devised this crossed-limb loop drainage catheter so that a nylon filament inside the catheter exits at the proximal hole and is attached to the catheter tip (A). Tension applied to the filament (B) causes the tip to bend backward and form a tight loop (C).

plastic anchoring suture was accidentally cut. To avoid such an accident, Cope covered the suture with a short section of rubber tubing.

The Improved CLL Catheter

In 1982, Cope improved the crossed-limb loop catheter by tying the suture to a point several centimeters proximal to the tip, as shown in Figure 11. As expected, tension applied to the suture caused a loop to form. However, because the suture was tied proximally, the loop closed and the distal part of the catheter projected at right angles to the catheter axis, as shown in Figure 11B. After inserting the catheter, Cope introduced a contrast agent and viewed the catheter fluoroscopically to assure patency of the drainage holes. He then glued a disk to the catheter about 2 cm from the skin to prevent forward migration; he did not need

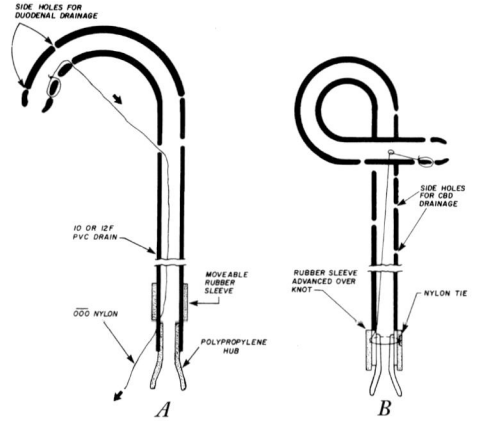

Fig. 11. In the improved crossed-limb loop drainage catheter, the nylon filament within the catheter exits at the proximal hole and is affixed a few centimeters back from the tip (A). Tension on the filament causes the tip to loop back and over the catheter.

to anchor it with skin sutures. Cope irrigated the catheter three times a week and replaced it every two months. Replacement was necessary because the vinyl loop became hardened if it remained in place longer than two months.

That same year Cope reported that hard concretions occasionally formed in the lumen of the CLL drainage catheter, making the catheter difficult to withdraw. To solve this problem, he attached a nylon suture, 40-cm long, to the proximal end of the catheter (Figure 12A). He then passed a Teflon sheath of the appropriate size over the drainage catheter and suture, as shown in Figure 12B. He held the suture with one hand and advanced the sheath with the other using a "twiddling" motion and forcing the loop to uncurl, as shown in Figure 12B.

Because of its reliable catheter retention qualities, the CLL drainage catheter, popularly known as the Cope Loop, was heralded as one of the most significant developments in drainage in the 1980s.

The Curved Dilating Catheter

Providing drainage for the biliary or upper renal system with a percutaneously inserted catheter first involved the insertion of a 22-gauge needle and injecting contrast agent through it to allow for fluoroscopic visualization. A slender guide wire was then passed through the needle to provide a path for insertion of a dilator to enlarge the tract. During this procedure, the slender guide wire often kinked, rendering the tract useless and often requiring more than one subsequent puncture with a larger needle to reach the desired site. In 1982, to provide a method that required only a single puncture to place the drainage catheter, Cope introduced a new instrument consisting of a stainless steel cannula and a 6.3-French curved Teflon catheter with a tapered tip.

Figure 13 shows the catheter assembly. An oval hole is located on the concave part of the catheter, just distal to the tapered tip. The tip is 3 cm long and

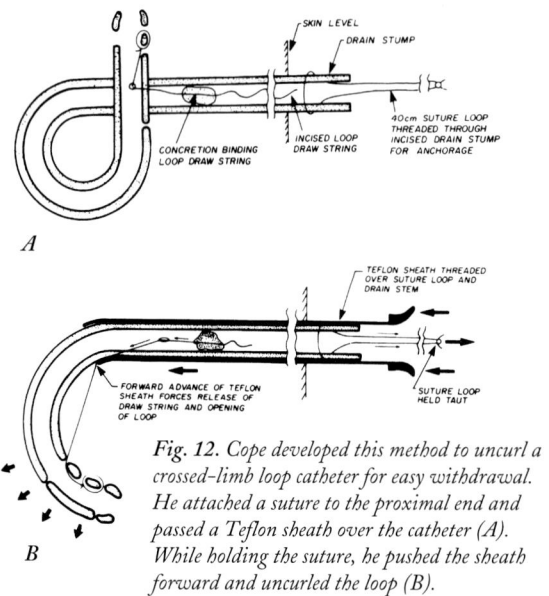

Fig. 12. Cope developed this method to uncurl a crossed-limb loop catheter for easy withdrawal. He attached a suture to the proximal end and passed a Teflon sheath over the catheter (A). While holding the suture, he pushed the sheath forward and uncurled the loop (B).

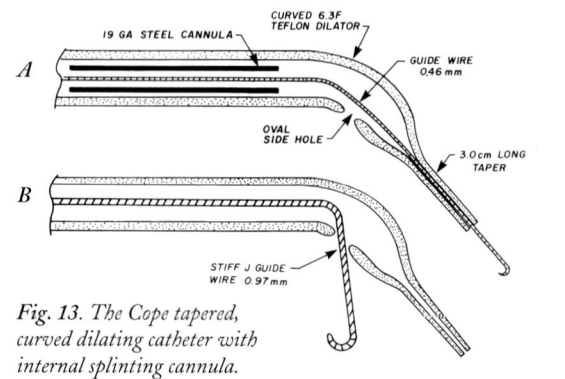

Fig. 13. The Cope tapered, curved dilating catheter with internal splinting cannula.

is tapered so that the lumen accepts an 0.53-mm guide wire. The oval hole is large enough to pass a 1.14-mm J guide wire freely. Note that this J-shaped guide wire is larger than the one that just filled the distal tapered lumen. The 19-gauge cannula can be placed inside the 6.4-French catheter and is long enough to reach the conical taper. The cannula provides a splinting action as the catheter is advanced through the tissue.

To establish the drainage tract, Cope advanced a 22-gauge needle to the target site and confirmed the location of the tip fluoroscopically using contrast agent. Then he passed an 0.46-mm guide wire through the needle and maneuvered it to the desired site. He replaced the needle over the guide wire with a 6.3-French curved Cope dilator catheter that was advanced under fluoroscopic observation using a gentle rotary motion to a depth of 6 to 7 cm. Cope paid out the catheter over the stiffening (internal) cannula until 3 to 5 cm of the thicker, nontapered portion was within the desired duct or space to be cannulated. The dilator catheter followed the fine guide wire without kinking, provided that the catheter was gently rotated while being advanced.

When the cannula and guide wire were at the desired site, Cope removed them and performed aspiration and/or irrigation. He threaded a stiff J guide wire into the catheter and maneuvered it easily so that it exited the oval side hole and entered the duct to be drained. Then he removed the 6.3-French dilator catheter, leaving the guide wire in place for further dilation.

Cope remarked that his dilator-cannula instrument was faster, simpler, and less traumatic than other methods, and he successfully demonstrated his claim in nephrostomies, biliary decompressions, and abscess decompressions.

Anchoring Device

In an effort to avoid leakage of fluid from a draining abdominal viscus, Cope devised a suture anchoring device. He actually developed two devices simultaneously. One is nonretrievable; the other "improved" version is retrievable. Both provided an effective seal against fluid leakage into the abdominal cavity.

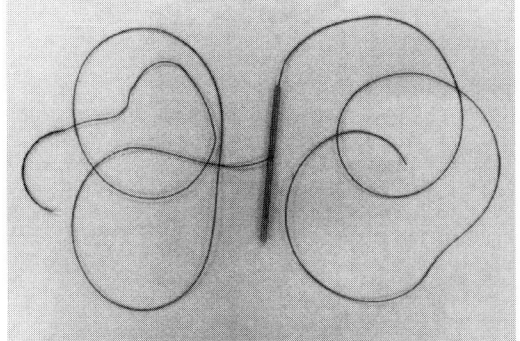

Fig. 14. Left: *The prototype retrieveable anchoring device developed by Cope.* Below Left: *(A) shows a suture passed into and out of the center of a short stainless steel crossbar, (B) the crossbar in the viscus, (C) the crossbar aligned at right angles to the catheter by pulling on the suture, and (D) the tilting of the cannula to permit removal.*

Cope's suture anchoring device (Figure 14) consisted of a stainless steel cannula, 6- to 10-mm long, into which he passed a suture that exited at mid-length (Figure 14A); these sutures were designated as end and center sutures. Using the conventional technique, Cope passed a cannula into the viscus and then passed the anchoring device into it, leaving the end suture trailing. He pushed the device along the catheter with a fine J-shaped guide wire until the guide's tip and the anchoring device entered the viscus (Figure 14B).

When he applied tension to the center suture, the crossbar aligned itself at right angles to the axis of the J guide wire and cannula (Figure 14C). He then tightened the sutures and secured them to the drainage catheter. He removed the anchoring device by tilting the cannula (Figure 14D) and cutting the end suture, thereby aligning the anchoring device with the cannula through which it exited.

Cope reported on his retrievable anchoring device in 1986, successfully draining the gallbladder and stomach without leakage and placing a catheter in the duodenum. His report prompted a great deal of interest, but the device is not yet commercially available. Fortunately for patients, the nonretrievable device (Cope Gastrointestinal Suture Anchor Set) is.

Fine-Needle Guide Wires

In 1983, Cope called attention to the fact that when an 18-gauge (or larger) needle was used to place a conventional guide wire to reach an obstructed cavity, a blood vessel or bowel wall might be lacerated. To eliminate that possibility, he proposed using a smaller, 22-gauge needle that necessitated a fine rigid mandrel wire (0.046-inch diameter, 60 cm long) tapered to a point along its distal 15 cm. Soldered to the tip was a coiled (0.46 mm) guide wire with a 6-mm J tip. Cope threaded this slender,

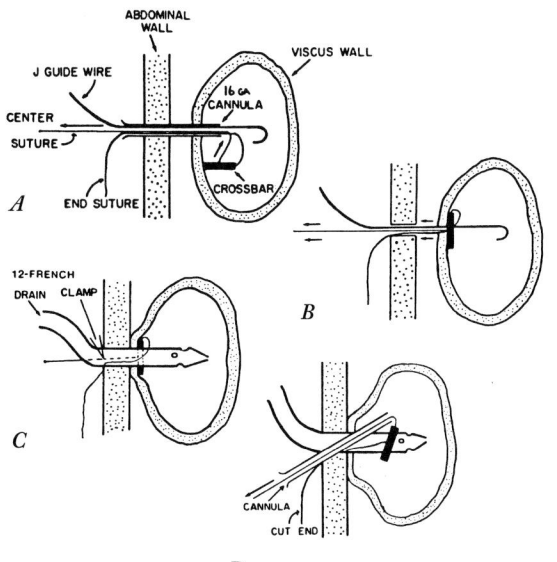

GOLDFINGER… COPE STYLE

Cope had to invent things that we take for granted. Early catheters were not radiopaque, so Cope placed gold rings on the tips and called the device "Goldfinger." (See Figure 15.)

Cope made his own catheterization kit, using items from gadget stores and assembling them in his kitchen. The kitchen location was fortuitous. When Cope tested his biopsy needle in the late 1950s, he worked with what was at hand. Biopsy-sized plugs were often missing from the fruits and vegetables in his family's larder.

Fig. 15. Cope's Goldfinger. *The gold rings on the tips of this catheter provide radiopacity, a precursor of modern techniques.*

stiff guide wire through a 22-gauge needle to reach the desired cavity and passed a 6- to 8-French catheter over the wire for drainage, thereby gaining access with a small initial puncture. Cope reported successful use of his fine-needle guide wire in thirty patients.

In 1983, Cope developed the Guidewire Exchange System, the first simple method of gaining access with a small needle, which ultimately led to the beginning of micro-puncture in the vascular system.

Cope's system included four components: (1) a 21-gauge needle; (2) a stainless steel guide wire with a helical coil J tip; (3) a 5-French dilator with a peel-away sheath specially tapered to fit snugly over the guide wire; and (4) a 6.3-French sheath dilator used to insert larger catheters. Cope successfully used this equipment to accomplish venous access via the subclavian, jugular, and internal jugular for hyperalimentation.

Cope said of the development of this procedure, "When I find a problem, I find that very exciting. It stimulates me to try to find a way to overcome or get around it. I like simple solutions, for that's the only way the technique is going to be useful."

Atlas Of Interventional Radiology

Cope, with his colleagues Burke and Meranze, compiled a vast array of interventional radiology techniques and in 1990 published the material in an impressive book, *Atlas of Interventional Radiology*. The volume includes many of Cope's devices and the techniques he uses in performing a variety of radiologic procedures. The atlas communicates the rationales, procedures, and results of his various interventions. An informative and practical tome, the book is aimed primarily at residents in radiology and fellows in training in interventional procedures. Surgeons and internists will find it valuable for acquainting themselves with the diagnostic and treatment modalities used by interventionalists.

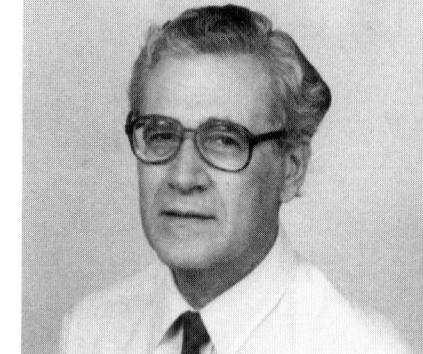

Fig. 16. Constantin Cope

According to Cope's comments in the preface, the success of interventional procedures depends not only on the innate knowledge and technical skill of the operator, but also on the operator's awareness of a variety of alternative approaches that can be selected in the course of managing a particularly difficult case.

A review in the July 1991 issue of the *American Journal of Roentgenology* suggested that Cope's atlas should be a part of every interventionalist's reference library. Glickman wrote:

"Heretofore, [Cope's] innovations have reached the medical community piecemeal in journals, at meetings, or in catheter company brochures. At last comes a book that shows the reader not just a series of clever wrinkles and intricate maneuvers but an overview of Dr. Cope's way of doing interventional radiology.

"It is a wonderfully satisfying book. Dr. Cope writes with a casual, common-sense directness and makes clear the why at the same time that he explains the how."

About Cope

Constantin Cope was born in Paris, France, on June 3, 1927. His parents had emigrated from Poland to Paris several years before. His father, Aaron Kopelowitz, was an engineer and may well have influenced Cope's creativity and love of gadgets. Kopelowitz was more perceptive than many Europeans of the time in believing that Hitler's rise to power posed the threat of mortal danger. In 1938, Kopelowitz fled Paris with his family and went to London, leaving much of what they owned behind.

After the blitz began, Constantin and his mother sought safety in the country near Cheltenham, England. Meanwhile his father traveled to New York on business and was stranded there when World War II broke out. As soon as possible after the war, Cope's mother left England to join her husband in New York City. At that time, the family shortened their last name to Cope.

Cope started his medical training at the University of London, where he received his Bachelor of Science and Bachelor of Medicine degrees, the latter in 1948. Then he transferred to New York Medical College to be closer to his parents, and he earned his M.D. degree in 1951. About this time, Cope started taking violin lessons and continued to study violin for about twenty years.

Following a medical internship at King's County Hospital from 1951 to 1953, he became a naturalized U.S. citizen. He then served as medical officer in the United States Army Medical Corps from 1953 to 1955, spending most of that time at an aid station on the front (truce) line in Korea. When he returned to the States, he took an internal medicine residency at West Haven Veterans Administration Hospital in West Haven, Connecticut.

In the summer of 1957, he married Mary Grace Heller from Englewood, New Jersey. After his marriage, he continued his training by taking a one-year residency in pulmonary diseases at East Orange Veterans Administration Hospital in East Orange, New Jersey. In the fall of 1958, Cope moved his family to Memphis, Tennessee, where he took a staff position in cancer chemotherapy at the Kennedy Veterans Administration Hospital. He was certified in internal medicine while in Tennessee.

Full-Time Angiographer

After two years in Memphis, Cope searched for a position as a full-time angiographer, but at the time hospitals had not yet envisioned establishing a full-time position in this relatively untried new subspecialty. In early 1963, Cope met the charismatic Renaissance man, Jacob Gershon-Cohen, at Albert Einstein Medical Center in Philadelphia. Dr. Gershon-Cohen gave Cope the opportunity he was looking for, and in the fall of 1963, the Cope family moved to Elkins Park, Pennsylvania. By then, Cope's family included two boys and one girl. One more son and daughter were born in Philadelphia over the next four years.

Constantin Cope, called Stan by his colleagues, has held a variety of professional appointments. He was head of the section of vascular diseases at the Albert Einstein Medical Center until 1986 and clinical professor of radiology at Temple University School of Medicine from 1980 to 1986. He is presently acting chief in the section of angiography and professor of radiology at the Hospital of the University of Pennsylvania. Cope is a member of ten medical and scientific societies and a fellow in three of them—the American College of Physicians, the College of Physicians of Philadelphia, and the Society of Cardiovascular and Interventional Radiologists.

At the time of this writing, his curriculum vitae lists eighty-two scientific papers; he was the senior author on most of them. He has written three book chapters in addition to being the senior author of the richly illustrated and comprehensive *Atlas of Interventional Radiology*.

Cope is a tireless tennis player. He also enjoys travel, music, and theater, and he reads for relaxation. All five of the Cope children settled in the Philadelphia area. Cope watches with pleasure as his seven (so far) grandchildren develop into potential tennis opponents. His constantly enlarging family provides a warm and bustling home environment.

Quiet and reserved by nature, Cope is reluctant to talk about his successes. However, he will explain that he was curious to see if he could find ways to improve diagnoses by less invasive techniques. He is somewhat bemused that his curiosity and his love of gadgets have made such a difference in the world of medicine.

Cope tells aspiring radiologists that now is a great time for them to make their marks because interventional radiology is experiencing an explosion of new devices and techniques. He encourages future radiologists to be innovative and implores them to consider a variety of techniques rather than rely solely on conventional methods.

However, Cope knows that such a unique perspective can only be gained from years of on-the-job experience. "Medicine is more of an art than a science," he says. "There are so many variables; it is very hard to predict how a procedure will work or how a disease will progress. Everybody is different, vessels are different, and people vary in their reaction to dye and insertion of catheters. That is where experience comes in."

THE COPE-COOK PARTNERSHIP

Constantin Cope and Cook have worked closely together since the early 1970s. This partnership spurred the development of a number of interventional products.

- Cook-Cope Type Loop, which was used in:
  Nephrostomy Sets
  Biliary Drainage Sets
  Catheter Extraction Sheaths
- Cope Catheter Introduction Systems
- Cope Gastrointestinal Suture Anchor Sets
- Micropuncture Introducer Sets

The partnership continues today, with several new interventional products in development.

Time Line

Year	Achievement	Contributor
1665	First recorded intravenous injection (into dogs)	*Wren* — Essentials
1667	First intravenous injections in a human	*Major* — Essentials
1667	First use of vascular catheters for blood transfusion	*Lower* — Essentials
1827	Needle and syringe developed to produce cataracts for practice surgery	*Neuner* — Essentials
1841	Forerunner of modern hypodermic needle and syringe introduced	*Jayne* — Essentials
1846	Urethra dilated by catheters of increasing diameters	*Benique* — Essentials
1850	First use of modern steel hypodermic needle and syringe	*Wood* — Essentials
1853	Experiments to coagulate blood with "Pravaz apparatus"	*Pravaz* — Essentials
1855	Development of balloon-tipped catheter for widening urethral strictures	*Reybard* — Essentials

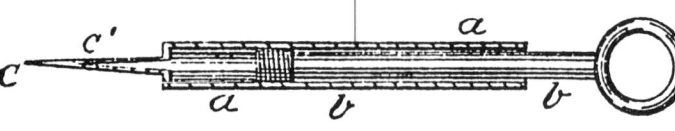

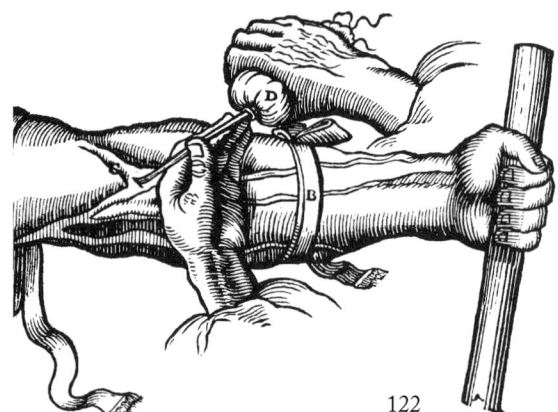

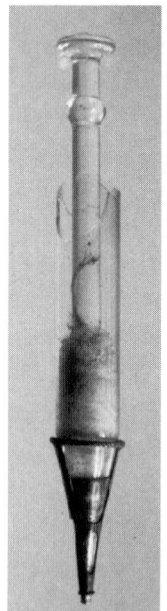

Legend
Achievement or event
Contributing individual or company
Chapter reference

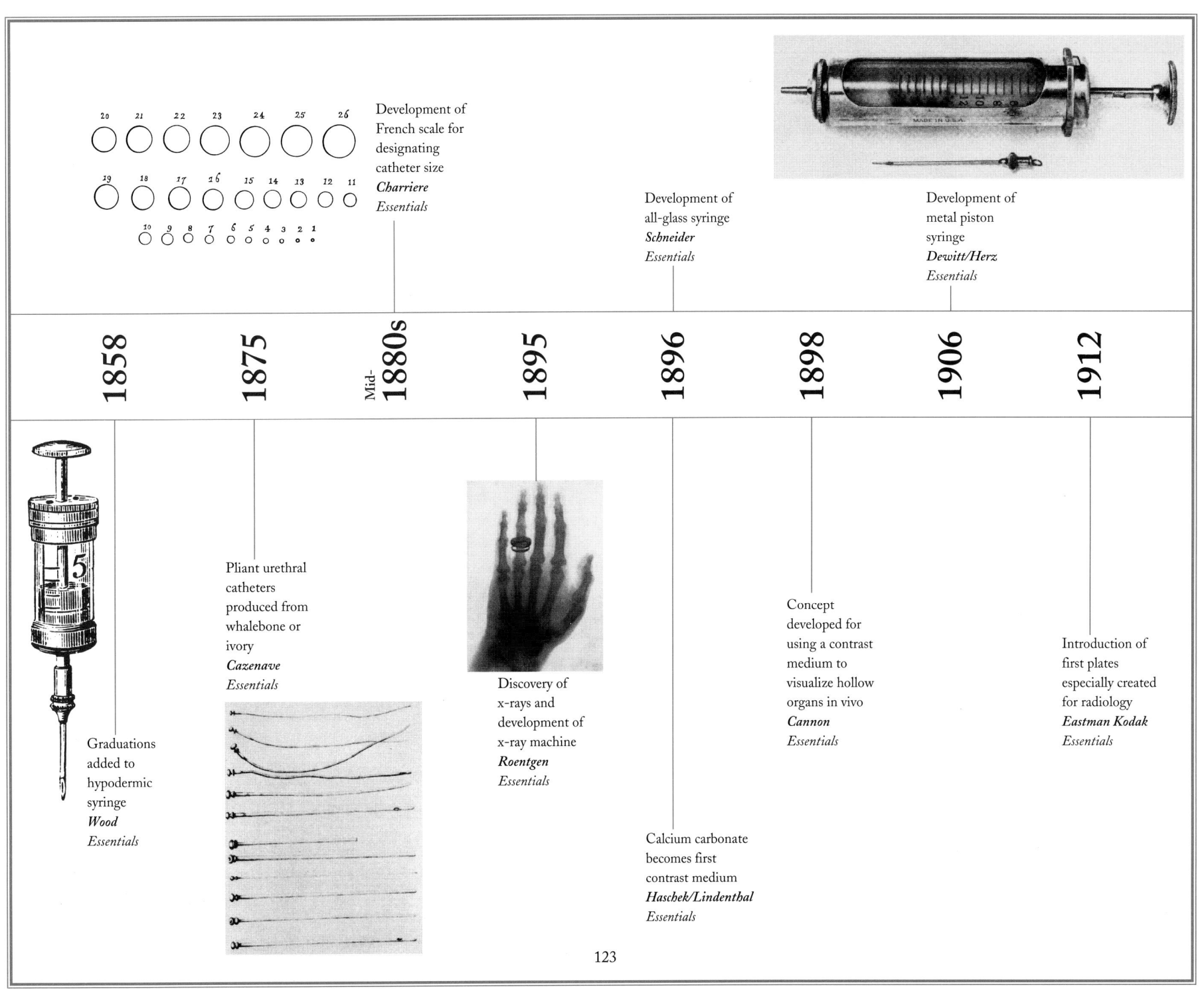

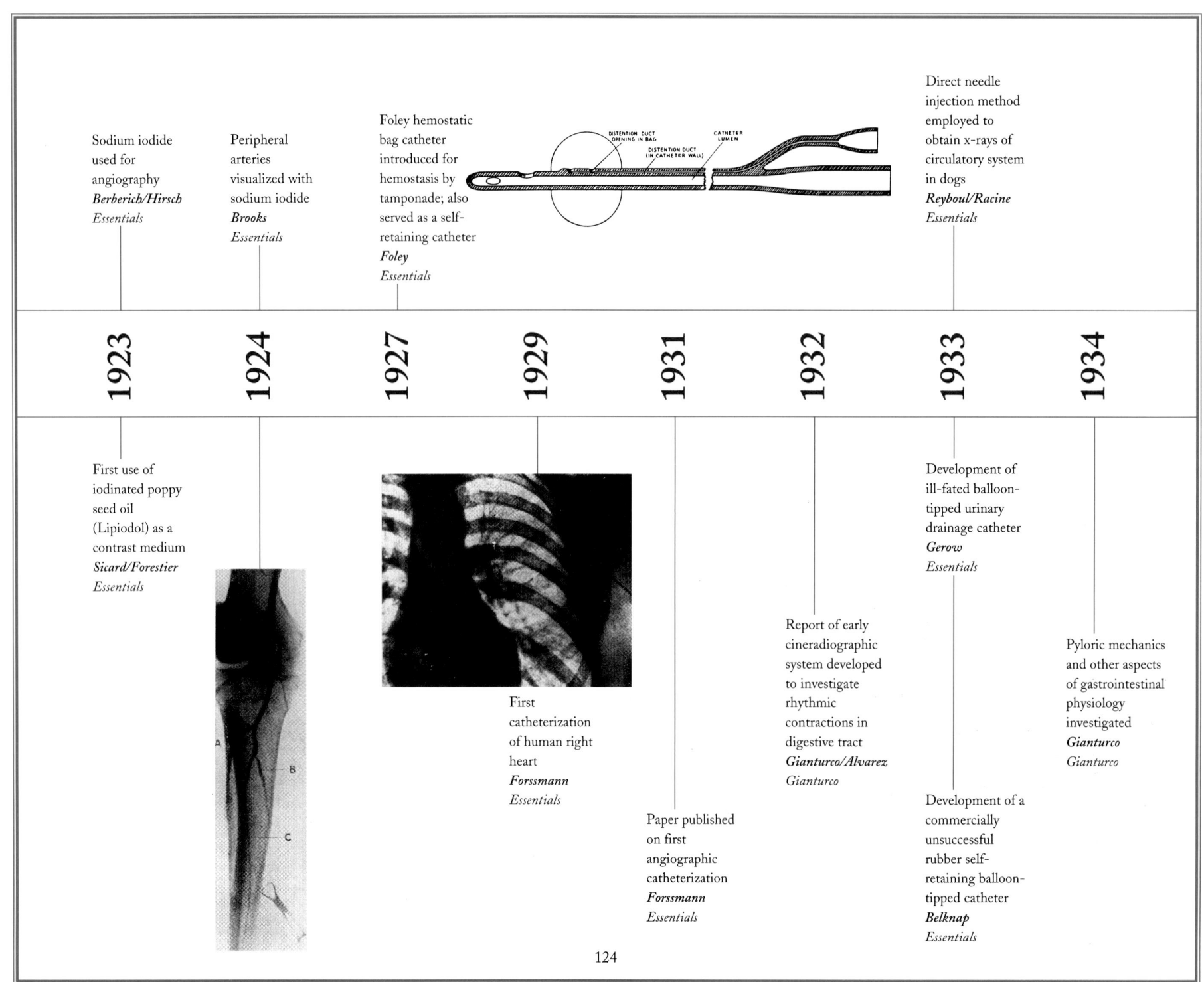

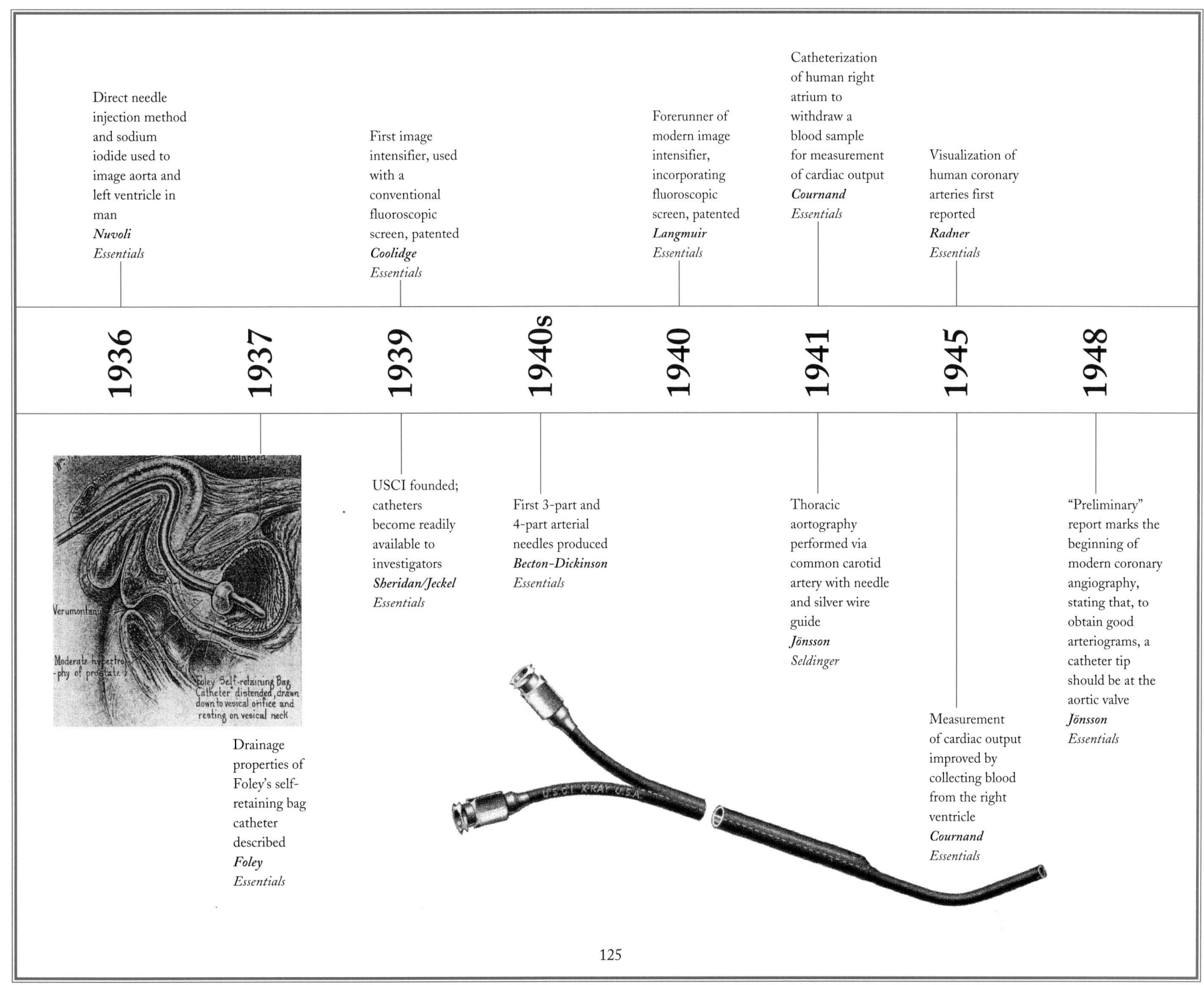

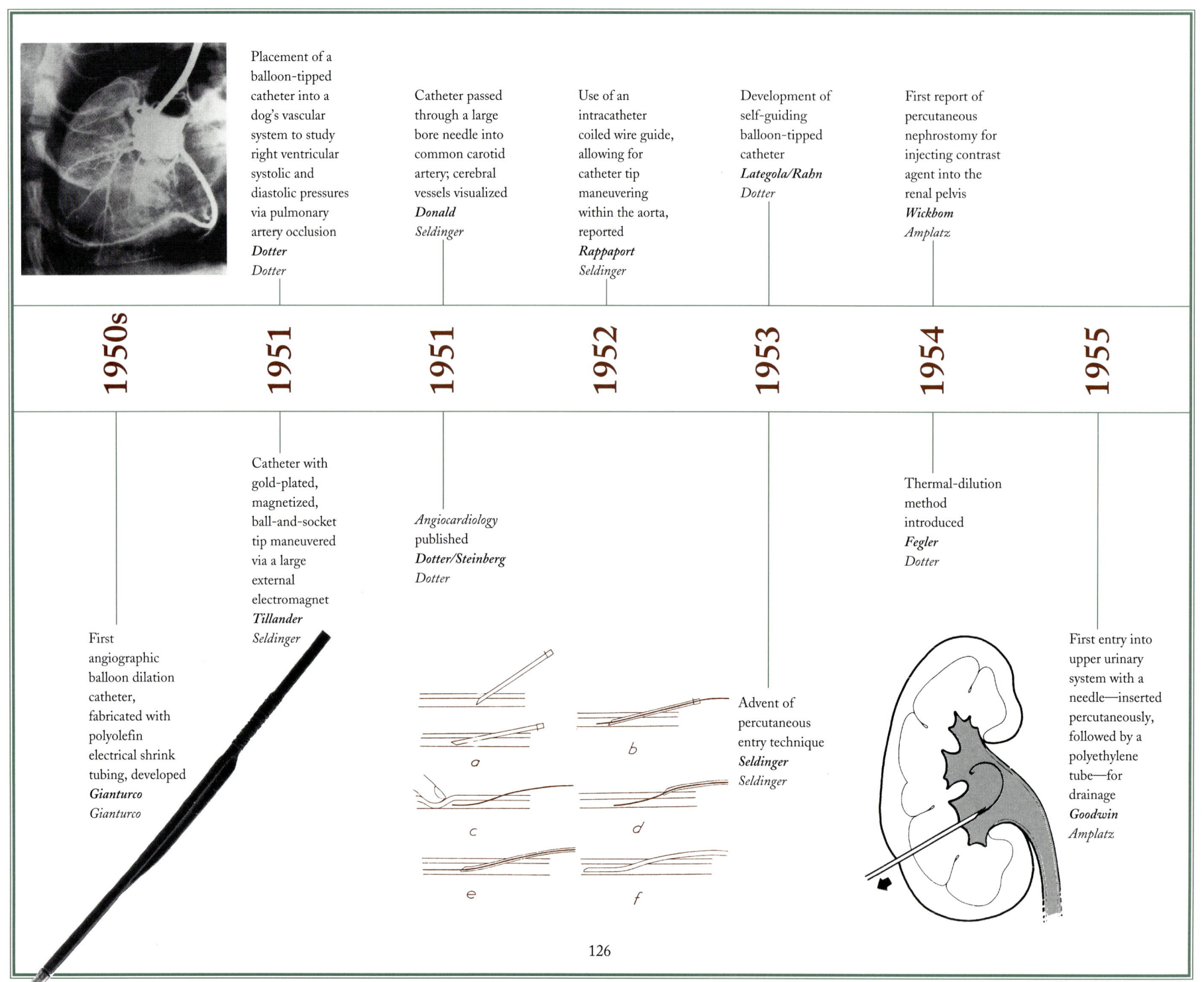

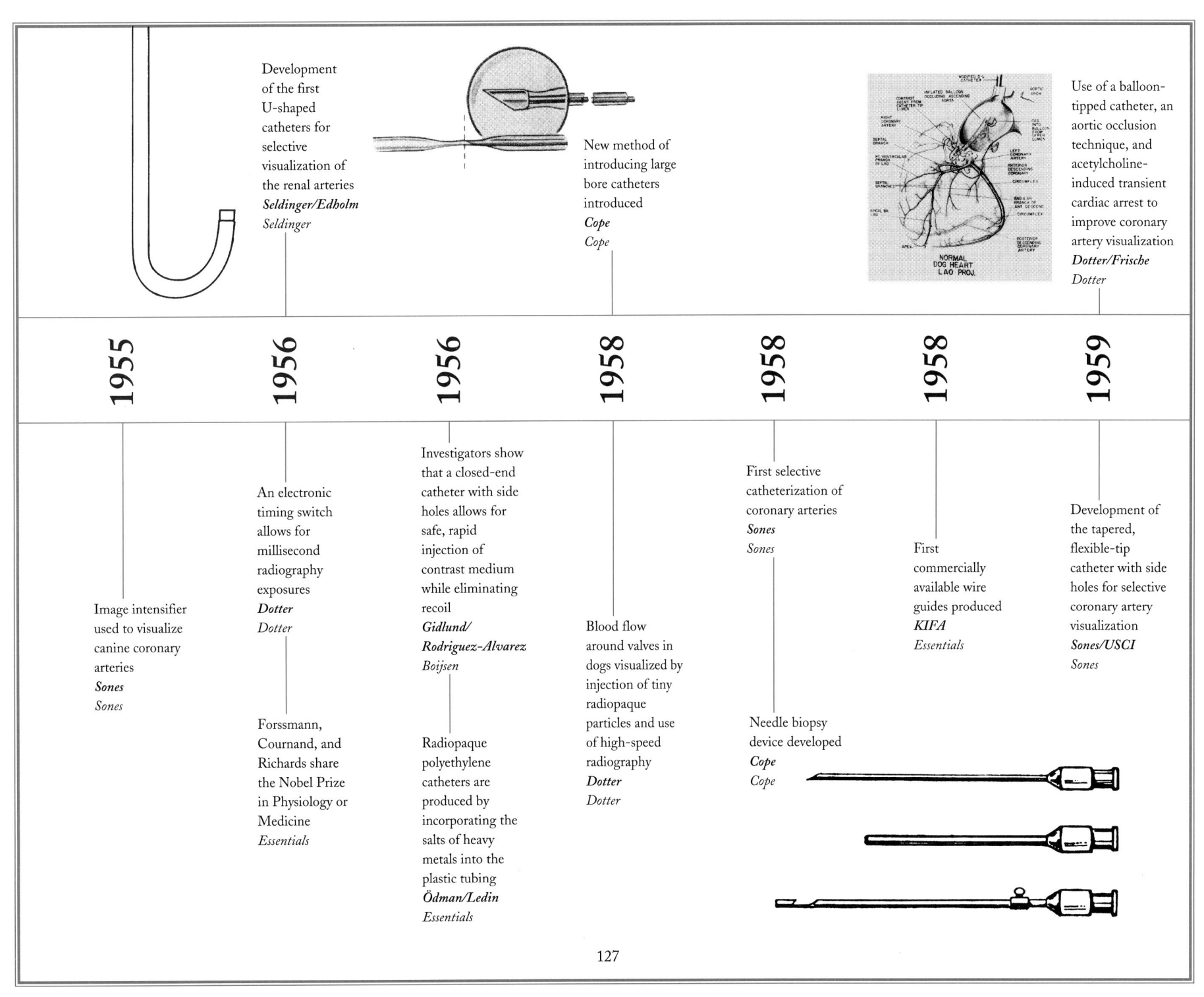

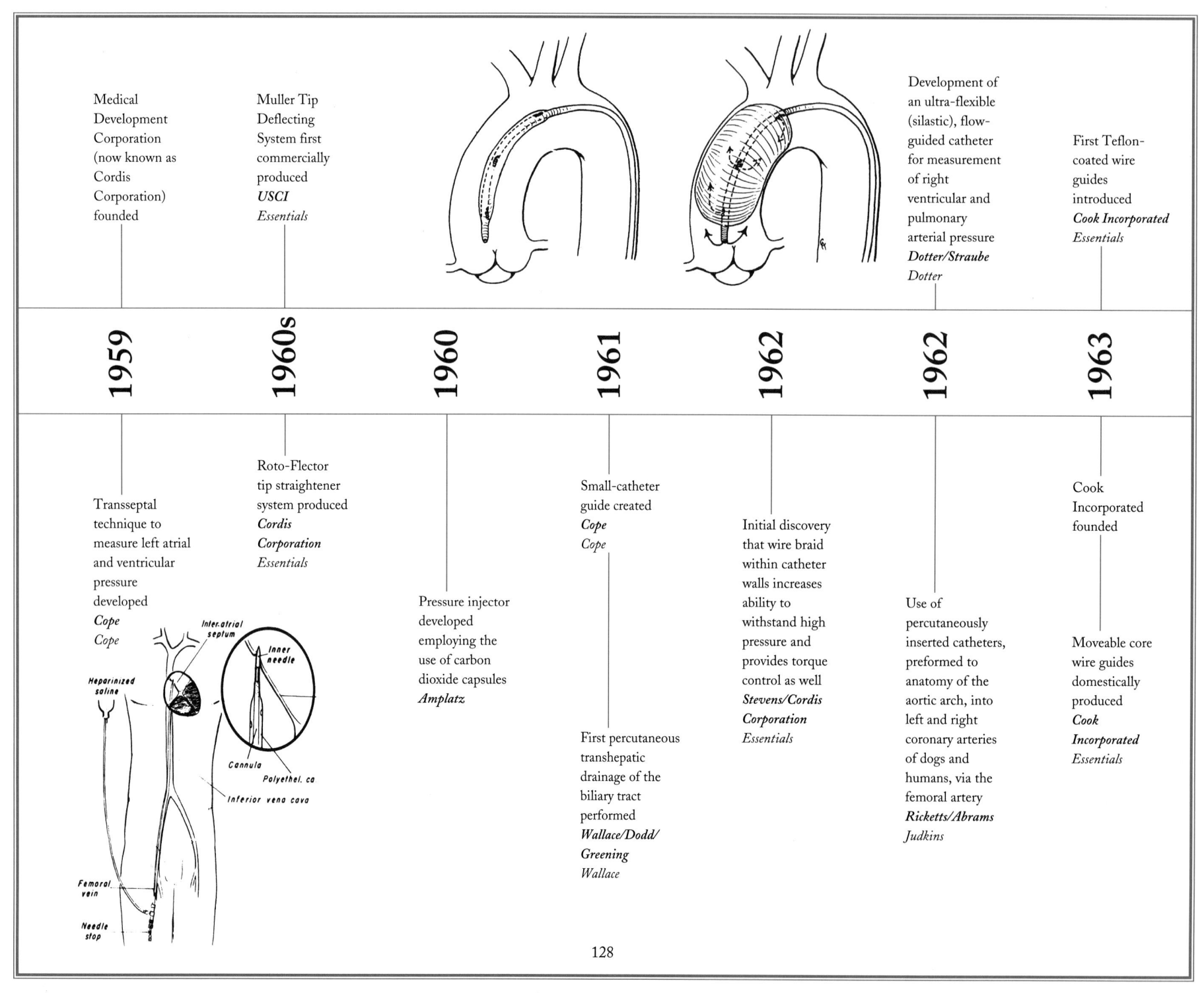

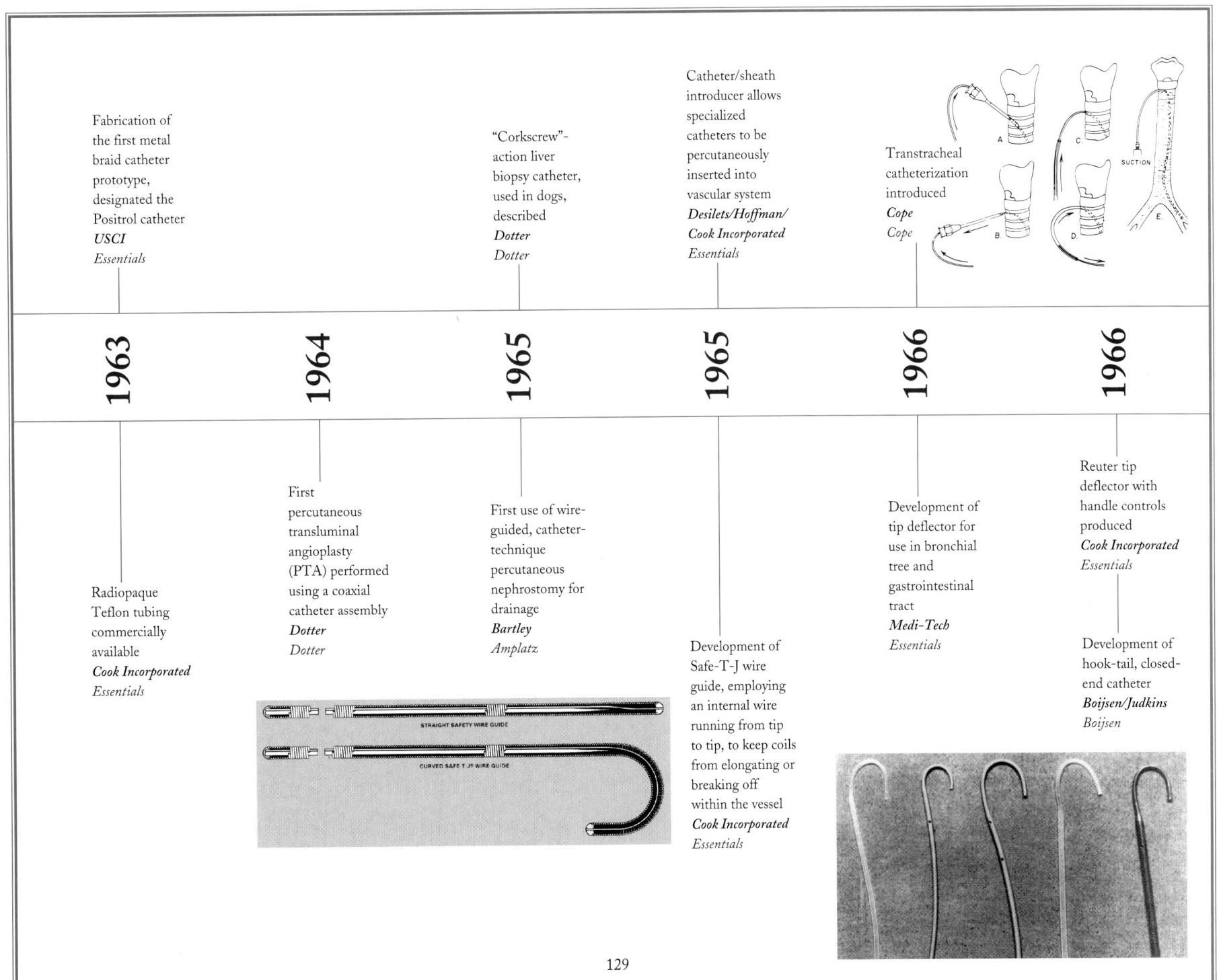

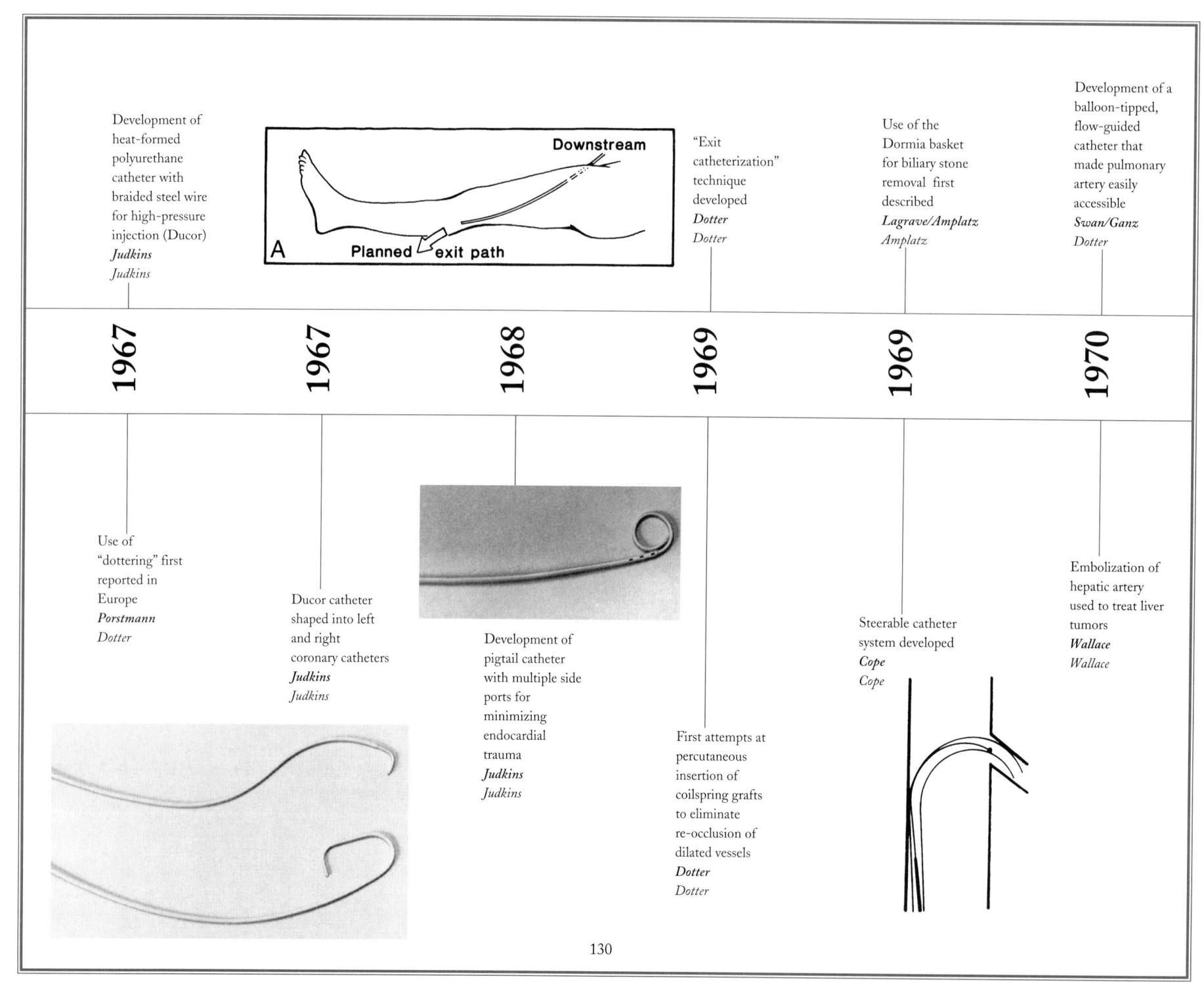

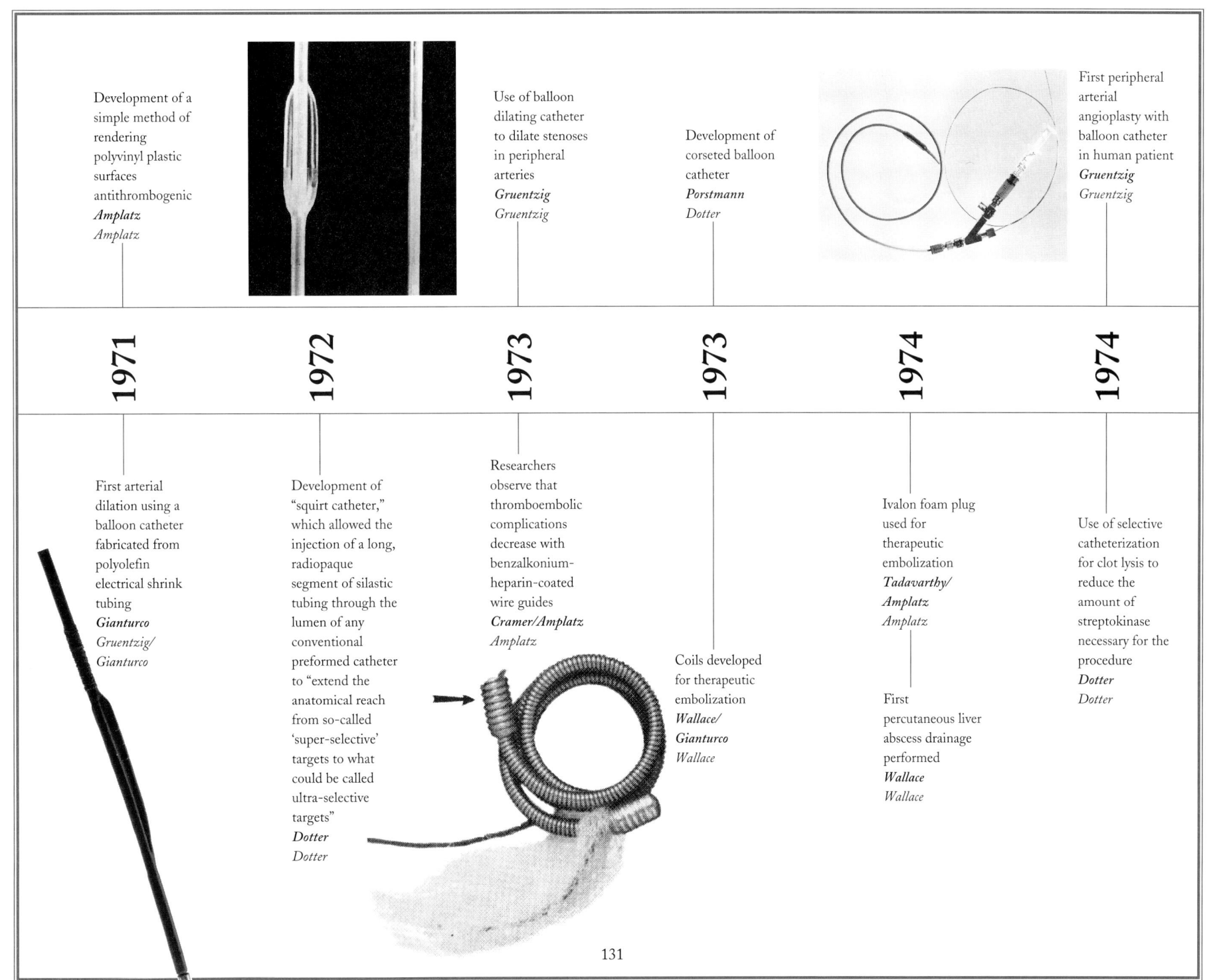

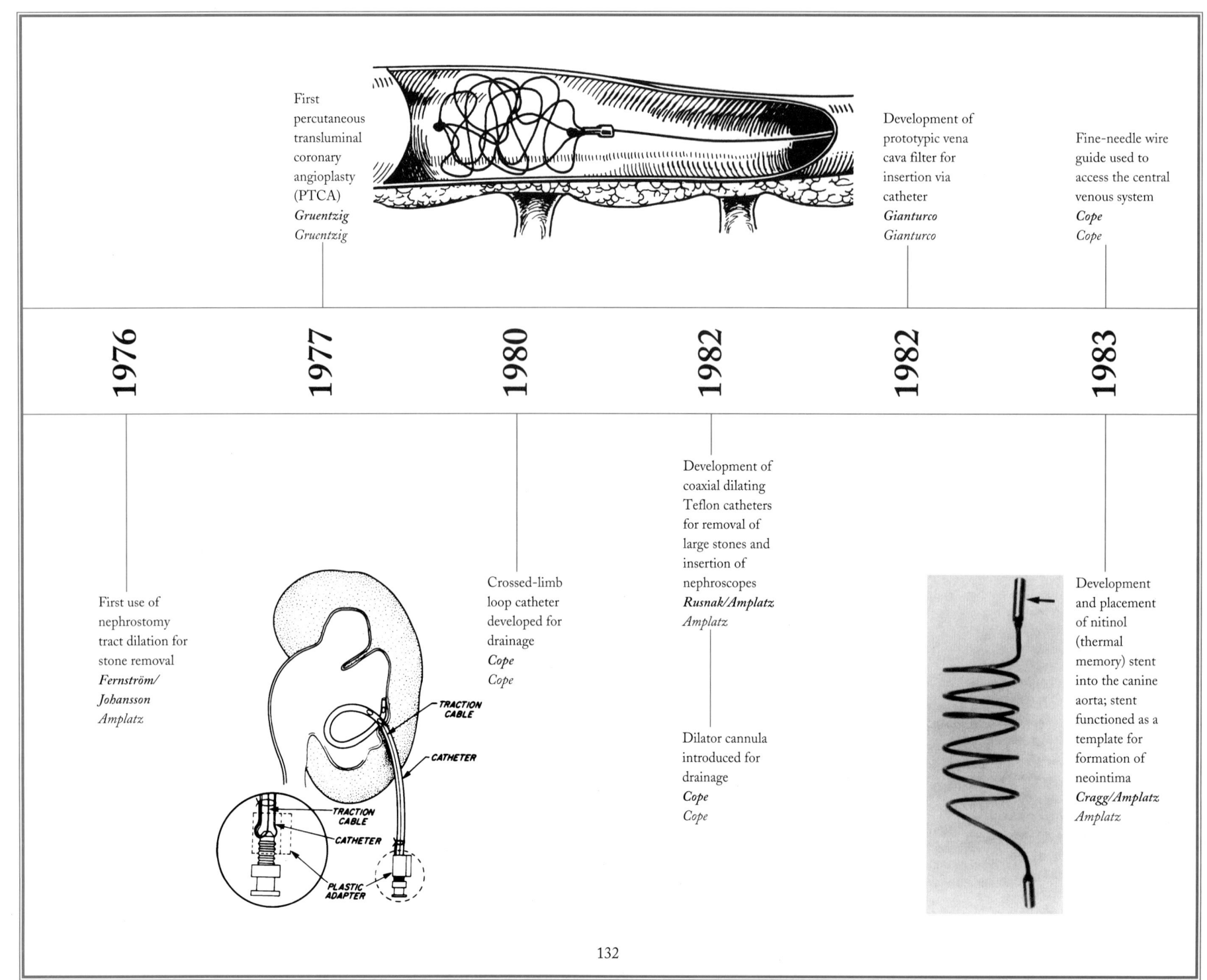

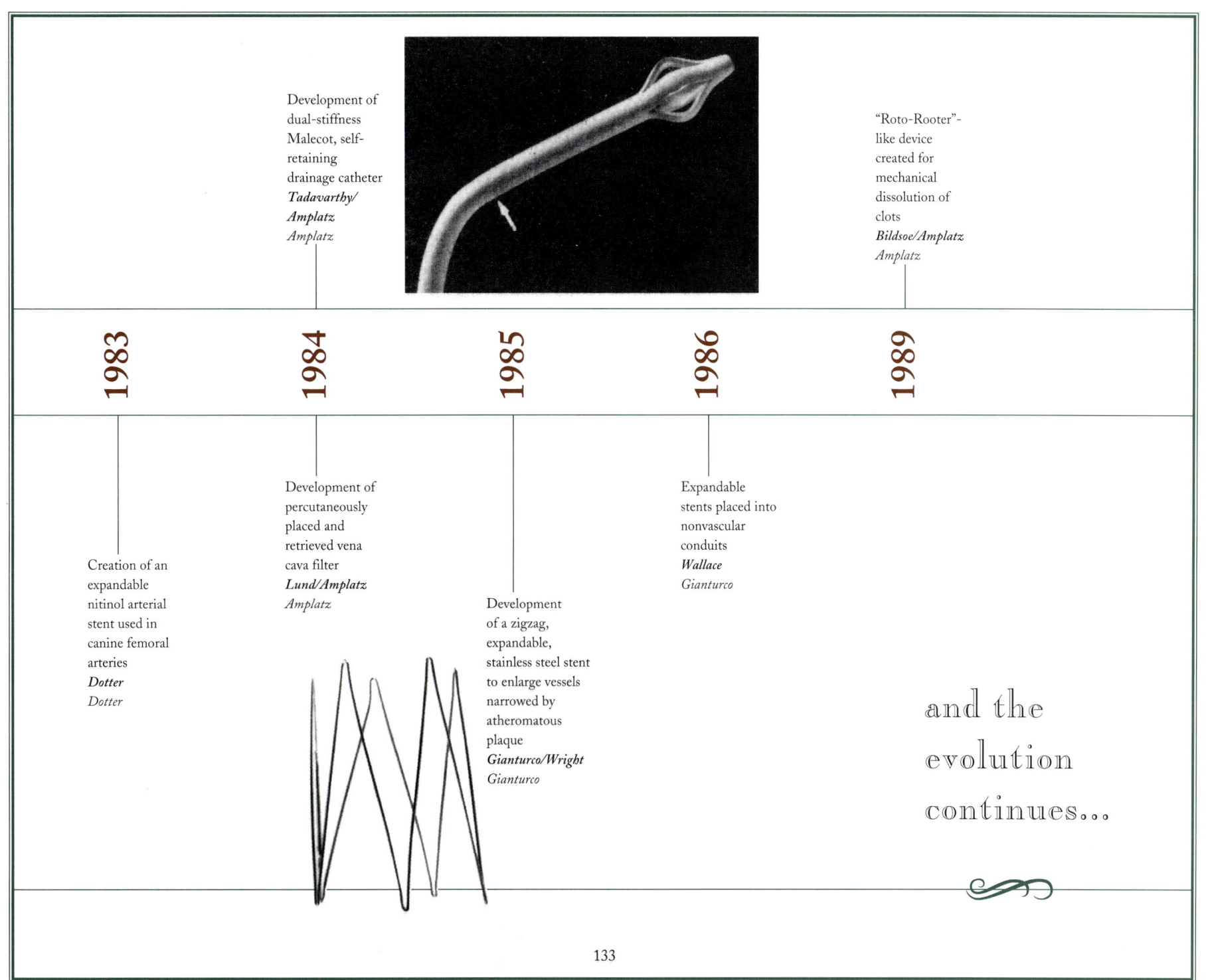

1983

Creation of an expandable nitinol arterial stent used in canine femoral arteries
Dotter
Dotter

1984

Development of dual-stiffness Malecot, self-retaining drainage catheter
Tadavarthy/Amplatz
Amplatz

Development of percutaneously placed and retrieved vena cava filter
Lund/Amplatz
Amplatz

1985

Development of a zigzag, expandable, stainless steel stent to enlarge vessels narrowed by atheromatous plaque
Gianturco/Wright
Gianturco

1986

Expandable stents placed into nonvascular conduits
Wallace
Gianturco

1989

"Roto-Rooter"-like device created for mechanical dissolution of clots
Bildsoe/Amplatz
Amplatz

and the evolution continues...

Notes on Contributors

Leslie A. Geddes

Leslie A. Geddes is professor emeritus at Purdue University in West Lafayette, Indiana. Until his retirement, he was the Showalter Distinguished Professor of bioengineering and director of the Hillenbrand Biomedical Engineering Center. Born in Scotland and educated in Canada, Geddes holds a bachelor's and a master's degree in electrical engineering 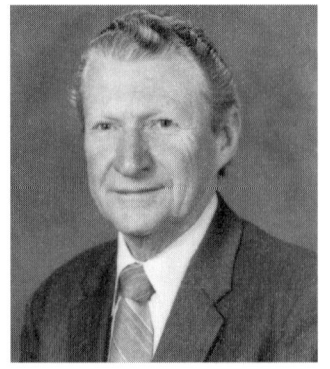 from McGill University in Montreal and a Ph.D. in physiology from Baylor University College of Medicine in Houston. He was awarded a D.Sc. Honoris Causa by McGill in 1971.

While at McGill, Geddes was an instructor in electrical engineering and in neurophysiology. While at Baylor, he was professor of physiology and director of the Division of Biomedical Engineering. Also while in Houston, Geddes was an adjunct professor of physiology at the University of Texas Dental Branch and at Texas A&M Veterinary College. He has conducted research in electromyography, cardiac output, cardiac pacing, ventricular defibrillation, blood pressure, and the properties of stimulating and recording electrodes.

Geddes and his colleagues have developed several new techniques for teaching medicine. He has written six books and more than five hundred scientific papers, receiving the Nightingale Prize for one paper and the Texas Medical Association award for a videotape on acute myocardial infarction.

Geddes is a member of numerous scientific societies; he is a fellow of the Institute of Electrical and Electronic Engineers, the American Association for the Advancement of Science, the American College of Cardiology, Australian College of Physical Scientists in Medicine, and the American Physiological Society. He is also affiliated with the Royal Society of Medicine. In 1985, he received the Alliance for Engineering in Medicine and Biology award for leadership in biomedical engineering, was elected to the National Academy of Engineering, and was the Rosenstadt Professor of Health Sciences at the University of Toronto. In 1986, he received the Institute of Electrical and Electronic Engineers/Engineering in Medicine and Biology Society Career Achievement Award and in 1987 the Association for the Advancement of Medical Instruments Laufman-Greatbatch award. In 1989, he received the Outstanding Educator award from the American Society for Engineering Education. He serves as a consulting editor to numerous scientific journals and is a consultant to the National Institutes of Health, the Food and Drug Administration, and the National Science Foundation.

Geddes is listed in *Who's Who in America, Leaders in the Southwest, American Men of Science,* and the *Royal Blue Book*. He is a naturalized United States citizen, is married to LaNelle (Nerger) Geddes, and has one son.

LaNelle E. Geddes

LaNelle E. Geddes was born in Houston and received all her formal education there. In 1957, she received a bachelor's degree in nursing from the University of Houston, and in 1970 she was awarded a Ph.D. in biophysics from the same institution. She served two years as a postdoctoral fellow in cardiovascular physiology at Baylor College of 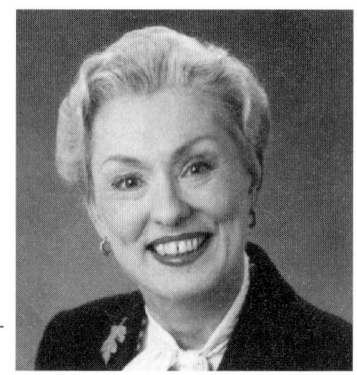 Medicine in Houston under a fellowship from the Division of Nursing, United States Public Health Service.

Geddes practiced medical-surgical nursing and school health nursing before entering the field of nursing education. During her teaching career, she taught graduate and undergraduate nursing students, served on numerous graduate committees, and provided both lecture and laboratory instruction for medical students, graduate students in fields outside of nursing, and fellows. She presented more than one hundred continuing education lectures and workshops to practicing nurses, other health providers, and members of the lay public. Throughout her academic career in research and teaching, she emphasized cardiovascular physiology and the impact of pathophysiologic alterations on the needs for nursing care.

Her honors and recognitions include citations in *Who's Who in America* and *American Men and Women of Science* and a number of teaching and leadership awards.

Geddes served as head of the School of Nursing from 1980 to 1991 and professor of nursing at Purdue University until 1992. She is now retired.

William A. Cook

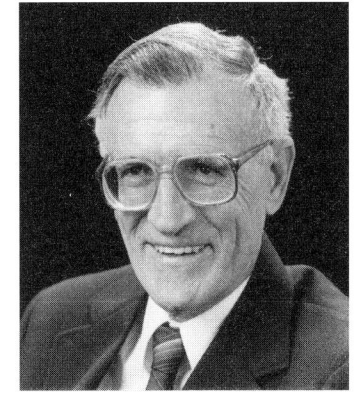

William A. Cook was born in 1931 in Mattoon, Illinois, and grew up in Canton, Illinois. He received a B.S. degree in 1953 from Northwestern University, Evanston, Illinois, with a major in biology. In May 1992, he received an Honorary Doctor of Engineering degree from Rose-Hulman Institute of Technology in Terre Haute, Indiana.

After serving as a medic in the U.S. Army, he worked as an engineering recruiter for Martin Aircraft and then as a catalog editor for American Hospital Supply Corporation. In 1958, in Chicago, he cofounded MPL Incorporated, a hypodermic needle manufacturing firm.

In 1963, Cook Incorporated was founded in Bloomington, Indiana, on $1,500 invested capital. Bill and his wife Gayle were the only employees. Percutaneous wire guides, catheters, and needles were the first products. The company has since grown into a conglomerate, Cook Group Incorporated, with manufacturing facilities in the United States, Australia, Denmark, Canada and, most recently, China. It has sales organizations around the world.

More than thirty companies form Cook Group Incorporated. The firms manufacture cardiovascular diagnostic and interventional products, extruded and injection-molded plastics, stainless steel tubing, pharmaceuticals, urologic equipment, pacemakers, OB/GYN devices, and endoscopic instruments. In addition, other Cook corporations are involved in real estate, electrical products, investment, retail fabrics, antiques, travel, charter buses, and aircraft service and leasing.

Cook has been instrumental in the restoration of many historic buildings in southern Indiana, including five properties on the National Register of Historic Places. He was a founder of the Monroe County YMCA, now the largest in Indiana, and is sponsor of the Star of Indiana Drum and Bugle Corps, a traveling and performing group of 128 young people. To aid the advancement of education and medical research, Cook companies provide significant financial support to universities, hospitals, and physicians throughout the country.

Cook has received numerous awards for achievement in community service, historic preservation, business, and medicine. He is a licensed jet pilot, has been the executive producer for nationally televised drum and bugle corps competitions, and has contributed to various books and periodicals. He serves as president and chairman of the board of Cook Group Incorporated.

Illustration References

Chapter 1

Fig. 1. Van Italie P. Rugged Beginnings of Injection Therapy, The Pulse of Pharmacy, Wyeth Co, 1965, 19[1].

Fig. 2. US Patent 2032, April 2, 1841.

Fig. 3. Reproduced by courtesy of the President and Fellows of the Royal College of Surgeons of Edinburgh.

Fig. 4. Howard-Jones N. The origins of hypodermic medication. Scientific American 1971;224:96-102.

Fig. 5. The Pulse of Pharmacy, Wyeth Co, 1965, 19[3].

Fig. 6. Courtesy of Cook Incorporated.

Fig. 7. Courtesy of Cook Incorporated.

Fig. 8. 1904 Wulfing-Lüer catalog, Paris.

Fig. 9. Reprinted by permission of the publishers from The Healing Hand: Man and Wound in the Ancient World by G. Majno, Cambridge, Mass.: Harvard University Press. © 1975 by the Presidents and Fellows of Harvard College.

Fig. 10. Reybard JF. Traite pratique des retrecissements du canal de l'uretre. Paris: Libraire de la Faculte de Medic, 1855.

Fig. 11. Lytton B. Perspectives in Urology. Nutley, NJ: Roche Laboratories, 1976.

Fig. 12. Redrawn from Lytton B. Perspectives in Urology. Nutley, NJ: Roche Laboratories, 1976.

Fig. 13. Reybard JF. Traite pratique des retrecissements de canal de l'uretre. Paris: Libraire de la Faculte de Medicine, 1855.

Fig. 14. Foley FEB. A hemostatic bag catheter. J Urol 1937;30:134-9. © by Williams & Wilkins, 1937.

Fig. 15. Foley FEB. A self-retaining bag catheter. J Urol 1937;30:140-3. © by Williams & Wilkins, 1937.

Fig. 16A. Thompson H. Clinical Lectures on Diseases of the Urinary Tract. Philadelphia: P Blakiston, Son, and Co, 7th edition, 1883.

Fig 16B. Lytton B. Perspectives in Urology. Nutley, NJ: Roche Laboratories, 1976.

Fig. 17. Forssmann W. Experiments on Myself. New York: St Martin's Press, 1972.

Fig. 18. Forssmann W. Experiments on Myself. New York: St Martin's Press, 1972.

Fig. 19. Courtesy of USCI.

Fig. 20. Courtesy of Siemens-Elema.

Fig. 21. Courtesy of Cordis Corporation.

Fig. 22. Courtesy of Cook Incorporated.

Fig. 23. Courtesy of Cook Incorporated.

Fig. 24. Schick X-ray, Chicago, IL. (defunct)

Fig. 25. Courtesy of Cook Incorporated.

Fig. 26. Courtesy of Cook Incorporated.

Fig. 27. Courtesy of USCI.

Fig. 28. Courtesy of Medi-Tech.

Fig. 29. Hodges PC. A visit to Roentgen's laboratory in 1923. Am J Roentgen Radium Ther 1946;56:642-6. © by American Roentgen Ray Society.

Fig. 30. Courtesy of the Burndy Library, Norwalk, Conn.

Fig. 31. Brooks B. Intra-arterial injection of sodium iodid. JAMA 1924;82:1016-9. © 1924 by American Medical Association.

Chapter 2

Fig. 1. Am J Roentgen 1984;142:5-7. © by American Roentgen Ray Society.

Fig. 2. Courtesy of Leslie and LaNelle Geddes.

Fig. 3. Seldinger SI. Acta Radiol 1952;39:369-76. © 1952 by Munksgaard International Publishers Ltd, Copenhagen, Denmark.

Fig. 4. Courtesy of Leslie and LaNelle Geddes.

Fig. 5. Edholm P and Seldinger SI. Acta Radiol 1956; 45:15-20. © 1956 by Munksgaard International Publishers Ltd, Copenhagen, Denmark.

Chapter 3

Fig. 1. Courtesy of Erik Boijsen.

Fig. 2. Boijsen E. A hook-tail "closed-end" catheter for percutaneous selective cardioangiography. Radiology 1966;87:872-7.

Fig. 3. Courtesy of Erik Boijsen.

Chapter 4

Fig. 1. Courtesy of Geraldine Sones.

Fig. 2. Courtesy of EK Shirey, MD, Cleveland Clinic.

Fig. 3. Courtesy of EK Shirey, MD, Cleveland Clinic.

Fig. 4. Courtesy of USCI.

Fig. 5. Courtesy of Cook Incorporated.

Fig. 6. Courtesy of USCI.

Chapter 5

Fig. 1. Courtesy of Eileen Judkins.

Fig. 2. Judkins MP. Percutaneous transfemoral selective coronary arteriography. Radiol Clin North Am 1968;6: 467-92.

Fig. 3. Judkins MP. Percutaneous transfemoral selective coronary arteriography. Radiol Clin North Am 1968;6:467-92.

Fig. 4. Judkins MP. Percutaneous transfemoral selective coronary arteriography. Radiol Clin North Am 1968;6:467-92.

Fig. 5. Judkins MP. Percutaneous transfemoral selective coronary arteriography. Radiol Clin North Am 1968;6:467-92.

Fig. 6. Courtesy of Eileen Judkins.

Chapter 6

Fig. 1. Courtesy of Cook Incorporated.

Fig. 2. Courtesy of Cook Incorporated.

Fig. 3. Dotter CT et al. Automatic roentgen-ray roll film magazine for angiocardiography and cerebral arteriography. Am J Roentgen Radium Ther 1949; 62(3):355-8. © by American Roentgen Ray Society.

Fig. 4. Dotter CT. Motion in cardiovascular radiography. Circulation 1955;12:1034-41.

Fig. 5. Dotter CT. Acute car pulmonale. Am J Physiol 1951;164:254-62.

Fig. 6. Dotter CT et al. Visualization of the coronary circulation by occlusion aortography. Radiology 1958;71(4):502-24.

Fig. 7. Straube KR, Dotter CT. Am J Roentgen Radium Ther Nucl Med 1963;90:650-4. © by American Roentgen Ray Society.

Fig. 8. Dotter CT, Straube KR. Flow guided cardiac catheterization. Am J Roentgen Radium Ther Nucl Med 1962;88(1):27-30. © by American Roentgen Ray Society.

Fig. 9. Reprinted with permission from The New England Journal of Medicine, 283, 447-51, 1970.

Fig. 10. Dotter CT et al. Injectable flow-guided coaxial catheters for selective angiography and controlled vascular occlusion. Radiology 1972;104(2):421-3.

Fig. 11. Dotter CT et al. Nonsurgical treatment of iliofemoral arteriosclerotic obstruction. Radiology 1966;86:871-5.

Fig. 12. Dotter CT et al. Transluminal iliac artery dilation. JAMA 1974;230:117-24. © 1974 by American Medical Association.

Fig. 13. Dotter CT. Exit catheterization. Am J Roentgen Radium Ther Nucl Med 1967;100(2):459-65. © by American Roentgen Ray Society.

Fig. 14. Dotter CT. Transluminally placed coilspring endarterial tube grafts. Invest Radiol 1969;4(5):329-32.
Fig. 15. Dotter CT et al. Safety coilspring for percutaneous cardiovascular catheterization. Am J Roentgen Radium Ther Nucl Med 1966;98:957-60. © by American Roentgen Ray Society.
Fig. 16. Dotter CT. Transluminal extraction of catheter and guide fragments from heart and great vessels. Am J Roentgen Radium Ther Nucl Med 1971; 111:467-72. © by American Roentgen Ray Society.
Fig. 17. Bilbao MK et al. Catheter retrieval of foreign body from the gastrointestinal tract. Am J Roentgen Radium Ther Nucl Med 1971;111:473-5. © by American Roentgen Ray Society.
Fig. 18. Dotter CT et al. Transluminal, expandable nitinol coil stent grafting: preliminary report. Radiology 1983; 147(1):259-60.
Fig. 19. Courtesy of Cook Incorporated.
Fig. 20. Courtesy of John Abele.
Fig. 21. Courtesy of the Radiological Society of North America.

Chapter 7
Fig. 1. Courtesy of Spencer B King III, MD.
Fig. 2. Courtesy of Ralph Lach, MD.
Fig. 3. Courtesy of Maria Schlumpf.
Fig. 4A. Zeitler E et al. Percutaneous Vascular Recanalization. Berlin: Springer-Verlag, 1978.
Fig. 4B. Courtesy of Maria Schlumpf.
Fig. 5. Zeitler E et al. Percutaneous Vascular Recanalization. Berlin: Springer-Verlag, 1978.

Chapter 8
Fig. 1. Courtesy of Kurt Amplatz.
Fig. 2. Amplatz K. A vascular injector with program selector. Radiology 1960;74:79-80.
Fig. 3. Redrawn from Amplatz K. Simple Bucky diaphragm for high speed angiography. Invest Radiol 1967;Nov-Dec:387-90.
Fig. 4. Redrawn from Amplatz K. New rapid roll-film changer. Radiology 1968;90:130-4.
Fig. 5. Amplatz K. A see-through 36 inch roll film changer. Am J Roentgen Radium Ther Nucl Med 1971;112(3): 628-9. © by American Roentgen Ray Society.
Fig. 6. Amplatz K. A new, simple test for thrombogenicity. Radiology 1976;120:53-5.
Fig. 7. Bildsoe MC et al. Mechanical clot dissolution: new concept. Radiology 1989;171:231-3.
Fig. 8. Cardella JF et al. Very stiff guide wire with a floppy tip. Radiology 1985;156:837.
Fig. 9. Smith T. Movable core guidewire. Radiology 1986;159:552-3.

Fig. 10. Butto F et al. New heavy duty exchange guidewire. Radiology 1987;163:276-8.
Fig. 11. Courtesy of Patricia Adams, The Johns Hopkins Hospital.
Fig. 12. Tadavarthy et al. Dual stiffness Malecot (Stamey) catheter. Radiology 1984;152:225. Smith et al. A new retention catheter. Radiology 1986;160:559-60.
Fig. 13. Courtesy of Cook Incorporated.
Fig. 14. Courtesy of Cook Incorporated.
Fig. 15. Lund G et al. Retrievable vena cava filter percutaneously introduced. Radiology 1985;155:831.
Fig. 16. Cragg A et al. Nonsurgical placement of arterial endoprosthesis: a new technique using nitinol wire. Radiology 1983;147(1):261-3.

Chapter 9
Fig. 1. Courtesy of Cook Incorporated.
Fig. 2. Gianturco C et al. Mechanical devices for arterial occlusion. Am J Roentgen Radium Ther Nucl Med 1975;124(3):428. © by American Roentgen Ray Society.
Fig. 3. Gianturco C et al. Mechanical devices for arterial occlusion. Am J Roentgen Radium Ther Nucl Med 1975;124(3):428. © by American Roentgen Ray Society.
Fig. 4. Courtesy of Cook Incorporated.
Fig. 5. Gianturco C et al. A new vena cava filter: experimental animal evaluation. Radiology 1980;137:835.
Fig. 6. Gianturco C et al. A new vena cava filter: experimental animal evaluation. Radiology 1980;137:835.
Fig. 7. Gianturco C et al. A new vena cava filter: experimental animal evaluation. Radiology 1980;137:835.
Fig. 8. Wright K et al. Percutaneous endovascular stents: an experimental evaluation. Radiology 1985;156:69.
Fig. 9. Duprat G et al. Flexible balloon-expanded stent for small vessels. Radiology 1987;162:276.
Fig. 10. Duprat G et al. Flexible balloon-expanded stent for small vessels. Radiology 1987;162:276.
Fig. 11. Uchida B et al. Modifications of Gianturco expandable wire stents. Am J Roentgen 1988;150(5):1185. © by American Roentgen Ray Society.
Fig. 12. Courtesy of Cook Incorporated.
Fig. 13. Courtesy of Cook Incorporated.

Chapter 10
Fig. 1. Wallace S. J Ark Med Soc 1981;77:479-86.
Fig. 2. Nealon T. Management of the Patient with Cancer, Vol III, WB Saunders Co, 1965;72-112.
Fig. 3. From J Microencapsulation, Vol 5, Wright K. Washington, DC: Taylor & Francis. Reproduced with permission.
Fig. 4. From J Microencapsulation, Vol 5, Wright K. Washington, DC: Taylor & Francis. Reproduced with permission.

Fig. 5. Anderson J. "Mini" Gianturco stainless steel coils for transcatheter vascular occlusion. Radiology 1979; 132:301-3.
Fig. 6. Wright K. Percutaneous endovascular stents: an experimental evaluation. Radiology 1985;156:69-72.
Fig. 7. Duprat G. Flexible balloon-expanded stent for small vessels. Radiology 1987;162:276-78.
Fig. 8. Courtesy of Cook Incorporated.
Fig. 9. Courtesy of Cook Incorporated.

Chapter 11
Fig. 1. Cope C. Simple method for introduction of large-gauge plastic catheters. Reprinted with permission from The New England Journal of Medicine, 258, 1000-2, 1958.
Fig. 2. Cope C. New pleural biopsy needle. JAMA Jan. 28. 1958;167;1107-8. © 1958 by American Medical Association.
Fig. 3. Cope C. Technique for transseptal catheterization of the left atrium. J Thor Surg 1959;37:482-6.
Fig. 4. Courtesy of Becton-Dickinson.
Fig. 5. Cope C. A new maneuverable guide for selective abdominal catheterization. J Appl Physiol 1961;16: 917-8.
Fig. 6. Cope C. Useful modification of the Cournand needle. Am Rev Respir Dis 1962;86:936.
Fig. 7. Cope C. Selective bronchial catheterization by a new percutaneous transtracheal technique. Am J Roentgen Radium Ther Nucl Med 1966;96:932-5. © by American Roentgen Ray Society.
Fig. 8. Cope C. A new safety device for retrograde power femoral arteriography. Radiology 1967;88:797-8.
Fig. 9. Cope C. A new one-catheter torque-guide system for percutaneous exploratory abdominal angiography. Radiology 1969;92:174-5.
Fig. 10. Cope C. Improved anchoring of nephrostomy catheter. Am J Roentgen 1980;135:402-3. © by American Roentgen Ray Society.
Fig. 11. Cope C. Use of crossed-limb loop anchor for percutaneous biliary bypass. Am J Roentgen 1982; 138:974-6. © by American Roentgen Ray Society.
Fig. 12. Cope C. Replacement of obstructed loops and pigtail nephrostomy and biliary drains. Am J Roentgen 1982;139:1022-3. © by American Roentgen Ray Society.
Fig. 13. Cope C. Conversion from small (0.018 inch) to large (0.038 inch) guide wires in percutaneous drainage procedures. Am J Roentgen 1982;138:170-1. © by American Roentgen Ray Society.
Fig. 14. Cope C. Suture anchor for visceral drainage. Am J Roentgen 1986;146:160-1. © by American Roentgen Ray Society.
Fig. 15. Courtesy of Constantin Cope.
Fig. 16. Courtesy of Constantin Cope.

References

Chapter 1

Abrams H, ed. Angiography. 2nd ed. 2 Vol. Boston: Little, Brown, 1971.

Allard EM. Sound and pressure signals obtained from a single intracardiac transducer. IRE Transactions on Bio-Medical Electronics 1962;9:74-7.

Almen T. Contrast agent design: some aspects on the synthesis of water soluble contrast agents of low osmolality. J Theor Biol 1969;24:216-26.

Amplatz K. A cardiovascular injector. Radiology 1960;74:79-80.

Amplatz K. A simple non-thrombogenic coating. Invest Radiol 1971;6(4):280-9.

Bean WJ, Mahorner HR. Removal of residual biliary stones through the T-tube tract. South Med J 1972;65:377-8.

Belknap HD. A new prostatic catheter bag. Urol Cutaneous Rev 1933;37:555-6.

Berberich J, Hirsch S. Die rintgenographische darstellung der arterien und venen am lebenden menschen. Klin Wochenschr 1923;49:2226-8.

Brannt W. India Rubber, Gutta-Percha, and Balata: Occurrence, Geographical Distribution...and Statistics of Commerce. Philadelphia: H.C. Baird, 1900:328.

Brooks B. Intra-arterial injection of sodium iodid. JAMA 1924;82:1016-9.

Cameron D. Aqueous solutions of potassium and sodium iodid as opaque mediums in roentgenography. JAMA 1918;70:754-5.

Cannon W. The movements of the stomach studied by means of the roentgen rays. Am J Physiol 1898;1:359-82.

Christophe L, Honoré D. L'artériographie par injection et prise de clichés automatiques. J Chir (Paris) 1947;63:5-11.

Chamberlain W. Flouroscopes and flouroscopy. Radiology 1942;38:383-413.

Coolidge W. The radiator type of tube. Am J Roentgen 1919;6:175-9.

Coolidge W. The development of modern roentgen-ray generating apparatus. Am J Roentgen Radium Ther 1930;24:605-20.

Cournand A, Ranges HA. Catheterization of the right auricle in man. Proc Soc Exp Biol Med 1941;46:462-6.

Cournand A, Riley RL, Breed ES, Baldwin E deF, Richards DW. Measurement of cardiac output in man using the technique of catheterization of the right auricle or ventricle. J Clin Invest 1945;24:106-16.

Diamond LK. A history of blood transfusion. In: Maxwell M. Wintrobe, ed. Blood, Pure and Eloquent: A Story of Discovery, of People, and of Ideas. New York: McGraw-Hill, 1980.

Dibner B. The new rays of professor Roentgen. Norwalk, CT: Burndy Library, 1963.

Eriksson JC, Gillberg G, Lagergren H. A new method for preparing nonthrombogenic plastic surfaces. J Biomed Mater Res 1967;1:301-12.

Farinas PL. A new technique for the arteriographic examination of the abdominal aorta and its branches. Am J Roentgen Radium Ther 1941;46:641-5.

Foley FEB. A hemostatic bag catheter. J Urol 1937;38:134-9.

Foley FEB. A self-retaining bag catheter. J Urol 1937;38:140-43.

Forssmann W. Experiments on Myself: Memoirs of a Surgeon in Germany. New York: St. Martin's Press, 1974.

Frank O. Kritik der elastischen Manometer. Z Biol 1903;44:445-613.

Gianturco C, Alvarez WC. Roentgen ray motion pictures of the stomach. Mayo Clin Proc 1932;7:669-71.

Gidlund A. Development of apparatus and methods for roentgen studies in haemodynamic. Acta Radiol [Diagn] (Stockh) 1956;Suppl 130.

Gouley JWS. Notes on American catheters and bougies. NY Med J 1893;58:85-8.

Grainger RG. Osmolality of intravascular radiological contrast media. Br J Radiol 1980;53:739-46.

Grainger RG. Intravascular contrast media—the past, the present and the future. Br J Radiol 1982;55:1-18.

Grode GA, Anderson SJ, Grotta HM, Falb RD. Nonthrombogenic materials via a simple coating process. Trans Am Soc Artif Intern Organs 1969;15:1-6.

Gross MJ, Atlee ZJ. Progress in the design and manufacture of x-ray tubes. Radiology 1933;21:365-77.

Grönbaum OFF. On a new method of recording alterations of pressure. J Physiol (Lond) 1897;22:xlix-li.

Guthrie GJ. On the anatomy and the diseases of the neck of the bladder and of the urethra. London: Burgess and Hill, 1834.

Haagensen CD, Lloyd WEB. Anaesthesia and Antiseptics. In: Ward H, ed. New Worlds in Medicine. New York: McBride, 1946:443-61.

Hales S. Statical essays, containing Haemastaticks. 2. London: W. Innys, R Manby and T. Woodward, 1733.

Hancock T. Personal Narrative of the Origin and Progress of the Caoutchouc or India-Rubber Manufacture in England. London: Longman, Brown, Green Longman, and Roberts, 1857.

Haschek F, Lindenthal OT. Ein beitrage zur praktischen Verwerthung der Photographie nach Roentgen. Wien Klin Wchnschr 1896;9(4):63-4.

Howard-Jones N. A critical study of the origins and early development of hypodermic medication. J Hist Med Allied Sci 1947;2:201-49.

Howard-Jones N. The origins of hypodermic medication. Sci Am 1971;224(1):96-102.

Hunter C, On narcotic injection in neuralgia. Med Times Gaz 1858; 2:408-9, 457-8.

Jönsson G. Thoracic aortography by means of a cannula inserted percutaneously into the common carotid artery. Acta Radiol [Diagn] (Stockh) 1949;31:376-86.

Jönsson G, Broden B, Karnell J. Selective angiocardiography. Acta Radiol [Diagn] (Stockh) 1949;32:486-97.

Lagergren H, Egberg N, Eriksson JC, Gillberg G. Preparation and evaluation of "nonthrombogenic" surfaces. J Thorac Cardiovasc Surg 1963;56:381-7.

Lambert EH, Wood EH. The use of a resistance wire, strain gauge manometer to measure intraarterial pressure. Mayo Clin Proc 1947;64:186-90.

Landes RR, Bush RB, Zorgniotti AW. Perspectives in Urology: the Official American Urological Association History of Urology. Nutley, NJ: Roche Laboratories, 1976.

Lindgren E. Technique of abdominal aortography. Acta Radiol [Diagn] (Stockh) 1953;39:205-18.

Lower R. An account of the experiment of transfusion, practised upon a man in London. Phil Trans Royal Soc (Lond) 1667;3(30):557-565.

Mahorner H, Bean WJ. Removal of a residual stone from the common bile duct without surgery. Ann Surg 1971;173:857-63.

Major JD. Chirurgie Infusoria, Kiel, 1667.

Marey EJ. La circulation du sang a l'etat physiologique et dans les maladies. Paris: G. Masson, 1881.

Mayno G. The Healing Hand: Man and Wound in the Ancient World. Cambridge: Harvard University Press, 1975.

Mazzariello R. Removal of residual bilary tract calculi without reoperation. Surgery 1970;67:566-73.

Mercier LA. Note sur de nouvelles sondes et bougies. Bull Natl Acad Med 1846;30:934-936.

Millar HD, Baker LE. A stable ultraminiature catheter-tip pressure transducer. Med Biol Eng 1973;11:86-9.

Murphy L. The History of Urology. Springfield: Thomas, 1972.

Moniz E. L'encéphalographie artérielle, son importance dans la localisation des tumeurs cérébrales. Rev Neurol (Paris) 1927;2:72-90.

Neuner A. Ueber die kuntsliche erlergung von cataraten in todten augen zum behuf der leichteren erlergung der staaroperationene. Chirurgie 1827;10:480-492.

Nuvoli. Arteriografia dell'aorta toracica mediante putura dell'aotra ascendente o del ventricolo. Polyclinico Sez Prat 1936;14:227-37.

Ödman P. The radiopaque polythene catheter. Acta Radiol [Diagn] (Stockh) 1959;52:52-64.

Ödman P. Thoracic aortography by means of a radiopaque polythene catheter inserted. Acta Radiol [Diagn] (Stockh) 45:117-24.

Osborne ED, Sutherland CG, Scholl AJ, Rowntree LG. Roentgenography of urinary tract during excretion of sodium iodid. JAMA 1923;80:368-73.

Poiseuille JLM. Recherches sur la force du coeur aortique. Paris: Didiot le Jeune; 1828. Thesis.

Ponsdomenech ER, Nunez VB. Heart puncture in man for diodrast visualization of the ventricular chambers and great arteries. Am Heart J 1951;41:643-50.

Potter HE. Diaphragming roentgen rays. Am J Roentgen 1916;3:142-5.

Pravaz CG. Sur un nouveau moyen d'operer la coagulation du sang dans les arteres. C R Acad Sci (Paris) 1853;36:88-90.

Radner S. Intracranial angiography via the vertebral artery. Acta Radiol [Diagn] (Stockh) 1947;28:838-42.

Reybard JF. Traite pratique des retrecissements du canal de l'uretre. Paris: Labe, 1853.

Reyboul H, Racine M. La ventriculographie cardiaque experimentale. Presse Med 1933;41:763-7.

Reynolds RJ. Cineradiography. Amer J Roentgen Radium Ther 1935;33:522-8.

Richards S, Thal AP. Phasic dye-injection control system for coronary arteriography in the human. Surg Gynecol Obstet 1958;107:739-43.

Robb GP, Steinberg I. A practical method of visualization of the chambers of the heart, the pulmonary circulation, and the great blood vessels in man. Am Soc Clin Invest 1938;17:507.

Rodriguez-Alvarez A. Am Heart J 1955;49:437-54.

Rodriguez-Alvarez A, Martinez de Rodriguez G. Studies in angiocardiography: the problems involved in the rapid, selective, and safe injections of radiopaque materials. Am Heart J 1957;53:841-53.

Seldinger SI. Catheter replacement of the needle in percutaneous arteriography. Acta Radiol [Diagn] (Stockh) 1953;39:368-76.

Sicard JA, Forestier G. Injections intra-vasculaire d'huile iodee sous controle radiologique. C R Soc Biol (Paris) 1923;88:1200-2.

Sovak M. Personal communication. La Jolla: Biophysica Foundation, 1987.

Stewart WH, Hoffman WJ, Ghiselin FH. Cinefluorography. Am J Roentgen Radium Ther 1937;38:465-9.

Thompson H. Clincial lectures on diseases of the urinary organs, delivered at University College Hospital, by Sir Henry Thompson. Philadelphia: HC Lea, 1869.

Thompson H. Clincial lectures on diseases of the urinary organs, delivered at University College Hospital by Sir Henry Thompson. Philadelphia: P Blakison, Son & Co., 1883.

Van Italie PH. Rugged beginnings of injection therapy. Pulse of Pharmacy 1965;19:3-6.

Viamonte M, Hobbs J. Automatic electric injector. Invest Radiol 1967:262-5.

Wetterer E. Eine neue manometrische sonde mit elektrischer transmission. Z Biol 1943;101:332-50.

Wintrobe MM, ed. Blood, Pure and Eloquent: A Story of Discovery, of People, and of Ideas. New York: McGraw-Hill, 1980.

Wood A. New method of treating neuralgias. Edin Med Surg J 1855; 82:265-281.

Wren C, comp. Parentalia; or, Memoirs of the Family of the Wrens. London: T. Osborn, 1750.

Chapter 2

Bierman HR, Miller ER, Byron RL Jr, Dod KS, Kelly KH, Black DH. Intra-arterial catheterization of the viscera in man. Am J Roentgen Radium Ther 1951;66:555-68.

Donald D, Kesmodel KF, Rollins SL, Paddison RM. An improved technique for percutaneous cerebral angiography. Arch Neurol Psychiatry 1951;65:508-10.

Farinas PL. A new technique for arteriographic examination of the abdominal aorta and its branches. Am J Roentgen Radium Ther 1941;46:641-5.

Jönsson G. Thoracic aortography by means of a cannula inserted percutaneously into the common carotid artery. Acta Radiol [Diag] (Stockh) 1949;31:376-86.

Peirce EC. Percutaneous femoral artery catheterization in man with special reference to aortography. Surg Gynecol Obstet 1951;93:56-74.

Radner S. Intracranial angiography via the vertebral artery. Acta Radiol [Diag] (Stockh) 1947;28:838-42.

Rappaport AM. The guided catheterization and radiography of the abdominal vessels. Can Med Assoc J 1952;67:93-100.

Seldinger SI. Catheter replacement of the needle in percutaneous arteriography. Acta Radiol [Diagn] (Stockh) 1953;39:368-76.

Edholm P, Seldinger SI. Percutaneous catheterization of the renal artery. Acta Radiol [Diagn] (Stockh) 1956;45:15-20.

Seldinger SI. Percutaneous transhepatic cholangiography. Acta Radiol [Diagn] (Stockh) 1966;Suppl 253.

Tillander H. Magnetic guidance of a catheter with articulated steel tip. Acta Radiol [Diagn] (Stockh) 1951;35:62-4.

Schobinger RA, Ruzicka FF, ed. Vascular Roentgenology; Arteriography, Phlebography. New York: MacMillan, 1964.

Chapter 3

Boijsen E, Judkins MP. A hook-tail "closed-end" catheter for percutaneous selective cardioangiography. Radiology 1966;87:872-7.

Boijsen E. Angiographic studies of the anatomy of single and multiple renal arteries. Acta Radiol [Diagn] (Stockh) 1959;Suppl 183.

Gidlund A. Development of apparatus and methods for roentgen studies in haemodynamics. Acta Radiol [Diagn] (Stockh) 1956;Suppl 130.

Rodriguez-Alvarez A, Dorbecker N. Studies in angiocardiography: the problem of injection. Am Heart J 1955;49:437-54.

Tornvall G. A modified catheter for percutaneous angiography. Acta Radiol [Diagn] (Stockh) 1957;47:470-2.

Nordenstrom B. New Instruments for catheterization and angiocardiography. Radiology 1965;85:256-9.

Olin T. Percutaneous introduction of tip-closed catheters. Angiology 1965;16:177-9.

Chapter 4

Arnulf G. L'arteriographie methodique. Soc de Chir, Lyon, 1958.

Bellman S, Frank HA, Lambert PB, Littmann D, Williams JA. Coronary arteriography. N Engl J Med 1960;262:325-8.

DiGugliemo L, Guttaduro M. On the radiological visualization of the coronary arteries in the living. Radiol Med 1954; 40(10):945-75.

Dotter CT, Frische LH, Hoskinson WS, Kawashima E, Phillips RW. Coronary arteriography during induced cardiac arrest and aortic occlusion. Arch Intern Med 1959;104:720-9.

Dotter CT, Lukas DS. Acute cor pulmonale: an experimental study utilizing a special cardiac catheter. Am J Physiol 1951;164:254-62.

Gordon AJ, Brahms SA, Sussman ML. Visualization of the coronary circulation during angiocardiography. Am Heart J 1950;39:114-24.

Grossman N. Visualization of the coronary arteries in dogs. Am J Roentgen Radium Ther 1945;54:57-9.

Haschek F, Lindenthal OT. Ein beitrag zur praktischen Verwerthung der Photographie nach Roentgen. Klinische Wochenschrift 1896;94:63-4.

Helmsworth JA, McGuire J, Felson B. Arteriography of the aorta and its branches by means of the polyethylene catheter. Am J Roentgen Radium Ther 1950;64:196-213.

Helmsworth J, McGuire J, Felson B, Scott RC. Visualization of the coronary arteries during life. Circulation 1951;3:282-8.

Horvath SM, Farrand A, Blatteis C, Everingham A. Catheterization of the coronary arteries of intact dog. Am Heart J 1957;54:138-45.

Hoyos JM, Gomez del Campo C. Angiography of the thoracic aorta and coronary vessels. Radiology 1948;50:211-3.

Hughes CR, Sartorius H, Kolff WJ. Angiography of the coronary arteries in the live dog. Cleve Clin Q 1956;23:251-5.

Lehman JS, Boyer RA, Winter FS. Coronary arteriography. Am J Roentgen Radium Ther Nucl Med 1959;81:749-63.

Jönsson G. Visualization of the coronary arteries. Acta Radiol [Diagn] (Stockh) 1948;29:536-40.

King SB, Douglas JS. Coronary Arteriography and Angioplasty. New York: McGraw-Hill, 1985.

Pearl F, Gray N, Friedman B. Retrograde aortography with a special catheter, including demonstration of the coronary arteries. Ann Surg 1950;132:959-64.

Radner S. An attempt at the roentgenologic visualization of the coronary blood vessels in man. Acta Radiol [Diagn] (Stockh) 1945;26:497-502.

Radner S. Thoracal aortography by catheterization from the radial artery. Acta Radiol [Diagn] (Stockh) 1948;29:178-80.

Richards LS, Thal AP. Phasic dye injection control system for coronary arteriography in the human. Surg Gynecol Obstet 1958;107:739-43.

Rousthoi P. Uber Angiokardiographie. Acta Radiol [Diagn] (Stockh) 1933;14:419-23.

Sones FM. Cinecardioangiography. In: Gordon BL, Kory RC, et al., ed. Clinical Cardiopulmonary Physiology. New York: Grune & Stratton, 1960.

Sones FM. Cine coronary arteriography. Mod Conc Cardiov Dis 1962;31:735-8.

Sones FM. Cine cardio arteriography. Anesth Analg 1967;46:499-508.

Sones FM. Cine-cardio-angiography. Pediatr Clin North Am 1958;5:945-79.

West JW, Guzman SV. Coronary dilatation and constriction visualized by selective arteriography. Circ Res 1959;7:527-36.

West JW, Kobayashi T, Guzman SV. Coronary artery catheterization in the intact dog. Circ Res 1958; 6:383-8.

Williams JA, Littmann D, Hall JH, Bellman S, Lambert PB, Frank HA. Coronary arteriography. N Engl J Med 1960;262:328-32.

Chapter 5

Adams DF, Fraser DB, Abrams HL. The complications of coronary arteriography. Circulation 1973;48: 609-18.

Baum S, Abrams HL. A j-shaped catheter for retrograde catheterization of tortuous vessels. Radiology 1964;83:436-7.

Boijsen E, Judkins MP. A hook tail "closed-end" catheter for percutaneous selective cardioangiography. Radiology 1966;87:872-7.

Dotter CT, Judkins MP, Frische LH. Safety guidespring for percutaneous cardiovascular catheterization. Am J Roentgen Radium Ther Nucl Med 1966;98:957-60.

Hinck VC, Judkins MP, Paxton HD. Simplified selective femorocerebral angiography. Radiology 1967;89:1048-52.

Judkins MP. Selective coronary arteriography. Part I: A percutaneous transfemoral technic. Radiology 1967;89:815-24.

Judkins MP. Percutaneous transfemoral selective coronary arteriography. Radiol Clin North Am 1968;6:467-92.

Judkins MP, Gander MP. Prevention of complications of coronary arteriography. Circulation 1974;49:599-602.

Judkins MP, Hinck VC, Dotter CT. Teflon-coated safety guides, an adjunct to the use of polyurethane catheters. Am J Roentgen Radium Ther Nucl Med 1968;104:223-4.

Judkins MP, Kidd HJ, Frische LH, Dotter CT. Lumen-following safety J-guide for catheterization of tortuous vessels. Radiology 1967;88:1127-30.

Judkins MP, Judkins E. Coronary arteriography and left ventriculography. In: King SB, Douglas JS, ed. Coronary Arteriography and Angioplasty. New York: McGraw-Hill, 1985.

Nebesar RA, Pollard JJ. A curved-tip guide wire for thoracic and abdominal angiography. Am J Roentgen Radium Ther Nucl Med 1966;97:508-10.

Ricketts HJ, Abrams HL. Percutaneous selective coronary cinearteriography. JAMA 1962;31:620-4.

Sones FM. Cine coronary arteriography. Modern Concepts in Cardiovasc Dis 1962;31:735-8.

Chapter 6

Bilbao MK, Bilbao J, Dotter CT. Lightweight medical kit for Alaskan expedition. Mazama 1968;50:20-4.

Bilbao MK, Kripphaene WW, Dotter CT. Catheter retrieval of foreign body from the gastrointestinal tract. Am J Roentgen Radium Ther Nucl Med 1971;111:473-5.

Dotter CT, Goldman ML, Rösch J. Instant selective arterial occlusion with Isobutyl 2-cyanoacrylate. Radiology 1975;114:227-30.

Dotter CT, Buschmann RW, McKinney MK, Rösch J. Transluminal expandable nitinol coil stent grafting: preliminary report. Radiology 1983;147:259-60.

Dotter CT, Judkins MP. Exit catheterization. Am J Roentgen Radium Ther Nucl Med 1967;100:459-65.

Dotter CT, Rösch J, Lakin PC, Lakin RC, Pegg JE. Injectable flow-guided coaxial catheters for selective angiography and controlled vascular occlusion. Radiology 1972;104:421-23.

Dotter CT. Transluminally placed coilspring endarterial tube grafts. Invest Radiol 1969;4:329-32.

Dotter CT, Rösch J, Seaman AJ. Selective clot lysis with low-dose streptokinase. Radiology 1974;111:31-7.

Dotter CT, Frische LH. Radiologic technic for qualitative and quantitative study of blood flow. Circulation 1958;18:961-70.

Dotter CT, Lukas DS. Acute car pulmonale. Am J Physiol 1951;164:254-62.

Dotter CT, Frische LH. Visualization of the coronary circulation by occlusion aortography: a practical method. Radiology 1958;71:502-24.

Dotter CT, Frische LH, Judkins MP, Mueller R. The "non-surgical" treatment of iliofemoral arteriosclerotic obstruction. Circulation 1964;30:654-70.

Dotter CT, Judkins MP. Transluminal treatment of arteriosclerotic obstruction. Circulation 1964;30:654-70.

Dotter CT. Transluminal angioplasty: a long view. Radiology 1980;135:561-4.

Dotter CT, Judkins MP, Frische LH. The non-surgical treatment of iliofemoral arteriosclerotic obstruction. Radiology 1966;86:871-5.

Dotter CT, Rösch J, Anderson JM, Antonovic R, Robinson M. Transluminal iliac artery dilation. JAMA 1974;230:117-24.

Dotter CT, Steinberg I. Automatic roentgen-ray roll-film magazine for angiocardiography and cerebral arteriography. Am J Roentgen Radium Ther 1949;62:3558.

Dotter CT. Motion in cardiovascular radiography. Circulation 1955;12:1034-42.

Dotter CT, Rogers TH. High-tension switch tube for roentgenography. Am J Roentgen Radium Ther Nucl Med 1956;75:83-90.

Dotter CT. Motion of blood-radiological studies. Third World Congress of Cardiology, 1956.

Dotter CT, Frische LH, Hoskinson WS, Kawashima E, Phillips RW. Coronary arteriography during induced cardiac arrest. Arch Int Med 1959;104:720-9.

Dotter CT, Straube K. Flow-guided cardiac catheterization. Am J Roentgen Radium Ther Nucl Med 1962;88:27-30.

Dotter CT. Intravascular tissue biopsy with a special catheter. Acta Radiol [Diagn] (Stockh) 1965;3:33-6.

Dotter CT, Rösch J, Bilbao MK. Transluminal extraction of catheter and guide fragments from the heart and great vessels: 29 collected cases. Am J Roentgen Radium Ther Nucl Med 1971;111:467-72.

Lategola M, Rahn M. A self-guiding catheter for cardiac and pulmonary arterial catheterization and occlusion. Proc Soc Exp Biol Med 1953;84:667-8.

Portstmann W. [A new corset balloon catheter for Dotter's transluminal recanalization with special reference to obliterations of the pelvic arteries.] Ein neuer Korsett-Ballonkatheter zur transluminalen Rekanalisation nach Dotter unter besonderer Berucksichtigung von Obliterationen an den Beckenarterien. Radiol Diagn 1973;14:239-44.

Portstmann W, Wierny L. Intravasle, rekanalization inoperabler arterieller Obliterationen. Zentralbl Chir 1967;92:1586-91.

Stevenson CA. Problems in radiology of today and the future. Am J Roentgen Radium Ther Nucl Med 1966;98:957-60.

Swan HJ, Ganz W, Forrester J, Marcus H, Diamond G, Chonette D. Catheterization of the heart in man with use of a flow-directed balloon-tipped catheter. N Engl J Med 1970;183:447-51.

Chapter 7

Belknap HD. A new prostatic catheter bag. Urol Cutaneous Rev 1933;37:555-6.

Dotter CT, Lukas DS. Acute cor pulmonale. Am J Physiol 1951;164:254-62.

Dotter CT, Frische LH, Hoskinson WS, Kawashima E, Phillips RW. Coronary arteriography during induced cardiac arrest and aortic occlusion. Arch Intern Med 1959;104:720-9.

Dotter C, Frische LH. Visualization of the coronary circulation by occlusion aortography: a practical method. Radiology 1958;71:502-24.

Dotter CT, Rösch J, Lakin PC, Lakin RC, Pegg JE. Injectable flow-guided coaxial catheters for selective angiography and controlled vascular occlusion. Radiology 1972;104:421-3.

Dotter CT, Lukas DS. Acute cor pulmonale Am J Physiol 1951;164:254-62.

Dotter CT, Frische LH, Judkins MP, Mueller R. The "nonsurgical" treatment of iliofemoral arteriosclerotic obstruction. Radiology 1966;86:871-5.

Dotter CT, Rösch J, Anderson JM, Antonovic R, Robinson M. Transluminal iliac artery dilatation. JAMA 1974;230:117-24.

Dotter CT, Judkins MP. Transluminal treatment of arteriosclerotic obstruction. Circulation 1964;30: 654-70.

Fegler G. Measurement of cardiac output in anaesthetized animals by a thermo-dilution method. Q J Exp Physiol Cognate Med Sci 1954;39:153-64.

Foley FEB. Cystoscopic prostatectomy: a new procedure and instrument. J Urol 1929;21:289-306.

Foley FEB. A hemostatic bag catheter. J Urol 1937;38:134-9.

Foley FEB. A self-retaining bag catheter. J Urol 1937; 38:140-3.

Ganz W, Donoso R, Marcus HS, Forrester JS, Swan HJC. A new technique for measurement of cardiac output by thermodilution in man. Am J Cardiol 1971;27:392-6.

Gruentzig A, Bollinger U, Brunner U, Schlumpf M, Wellauer J. Dotter's percutaneous recanalization in chronic arterial occlusions—a nonsurgical catheter technic. Schwiez Med Wochenschr 1973;103:825-31.

Gruentzig A, Hopff H. Percutaneous recanalization after chronic arterial occlusion with a new dilator-catheter (modification of the Dotter technique). Dtsch Med Wochenschr 1974;99:2502-10.

Gruentzig A, Senning A, Siegenthaler WE. Nonoperative dilation of coronary-artery stenosis. N Engl J Med 1979;301:61-8.

Gruentzig A. Transluminal dilation of coronary-artery stenosis (letter to editor). Lancet 1978;1(8058):263.

Gruentzig A. Die perkutante Rekanalisation chronischer arterieller Verschlusse (Dotter-Prinzip) mit einem meuen doppellumigeh Dilationskatheter forts. Geb Roentgen Nuklear-med 1976;124:80-6.

Gruentzig A. Die perkutane transluminale Rekanalisation chronischer Arterienverschlusse mit einer neuen Dilatationstechnik. Baden-Baden: Witzstrock, 1977.

Hurst JW. The first coronary angioplasty as described by Andreas Gruentzig. Am J Cardiol 1986;57:185-6.

King SB, Douglas JS. Coronary Arteriography and Angioplasty. New York: McGraw-Hill, 1985.

Lategola M, Rahn M. A self-guiding catheter for cardiac and pulmonary arterial catheterization and occlusion. Proc Soc Exp Biol Med 1953;84:667-8.

Porstmann W. [A new corset balloon catheter for Dotter's transluminal recanalization with special reference to obliterations of the pelvic arteries.] Ein neuer Korsett-Ballonkatheter zur transluminalen Rekanalisation nach Dotter unter besonderer Berucksichtigung von Obliterationen an den Beckenarterien. Radiol Diagn 1973;14:239-44.

Straube KR, Dotter CT. Single lumen balloon catheter for percutaneous insertion. Am J Roentgen Radium Ther Nucl Med 1963;90:650-4.

Swan HJC, Ganz W, Forrester J, Marcus H, Diamond G, Chonette D. Cardiac catheterization with a flow-directed balloon-tipped catheter. N Engl J Med 1970;283:447-51.

Zeitler E, Gruentzig A, Schoop W, ed. Percutaneous Vascular Recanalization. Berlin: Springer-Verlag, 1978.

Chapter 8

Amplatz K. New rapid roll-film changer. Radiology 1968; 90:130-4.

Amplatz K. Automatic injection syringe and cassette changer for cerebral angiography. JAMA 1963;183:430-3.

Amplatz K. Simple Bucky diaphragm for high speed angiography. Invest Radiol 1967;2:387-90.

Amplatz K. A see-through 36 inch roll film changer. Am J Roentgen Radium Ther Nucl Med 1971;112:628-30.

Amplatz K. A cardiovascular injector. Radiology 1960; 74:79-80.

Amplatz K. A vascular injector with program selector. Radiology 1960;75(6):955-6.

Amplatz K. Disposable catheter needles. Invest Radiol 1966;1:262-3.

Amplatz K. A new, simple test for thrombogenicity. Radiology 1976;120:53-5.

Amplatz K. A simple, non-thrombogenic coating. Invest Radiol 1971;6:280-9.

Bartley O, Chidekel N, Rüdberg C. Percutaneous drainage of the renal pelvis for uraemia due to obstructed urinary outflow. Acta Chir Scand 1964;129:443-6.

Bildsoe MC, Moradian GP, Hunter DW, Castaneda-Zuniga WR, Amplatz K. Mechanical clot dissolution: new concept. Radiology 1989;171:231-3.

Butto F, Robinson JD, Hunter DW, Castaneda-Zuniga WR, Amplatz K. New heavy duty exchange guide wire. Radiology 1987;163:276-8.

Cardella JF, Castaneda-Zuniga WR, Hunter DW, Young AT, Amplatz K. A new pyeloureteral drainage catheter. Radiology 1985;155:527-8.

Cardella JF, Kotula F, Hunter DW, Young AT, Casteneda-Zuniga WR, Amplatz K. Very stiff guide wire with a floppy tip. Radiology 1985;156:837.

Castaneda-Zuniga WR, Amplatz K, Laerum F, Formanek A, Sibley R, Vlodaver Z. Mechanisms of angioplasty: and experimental approach. RadioGraphics 1981;1(3):1-14.

Castaneda-Zuniga WR, Formanek A, Tadavarthy M, Vlodaver Z, Edwards JE, Zollikofer C et al. The mechanism of balloon angioplasty. Radiology 1980;135:565-71.

Castaneda F, Reddy PK, Hulbert JC, Lund G, Letourneau JG, Wasserman N et al. Retrograde prostatic urethroplasty with a balloon catheter. Seminars in Intervent Radiol 1987;4(2):115-21.

Castaneda-Zuniga WR, Clayman R, Smith A, Rusnak B, Herrera M, Amplatz K. Nephrostolithotomy: percutaneous techiques for urinary calculus removal. Am J Roentgen 1982;139:721-6.

Castaneda-Zuniga WR, Amplatz K. Percutaneous nephrostomy with the Stamey catheter: a new introducing technique. Urol Clin North Am 1982;9:65-7.

Castaneda-Zuniga W, Zollikofer C, Barreto A, Formanek A, Amplatz K. A new device for the safe delivery of stainless steel coils. Radiology 1980;230-1.

Coleman CC, Clayman RV, Lange PH, Castaneda-Zuniga WR, Miller R, Reddy P et al. Percutaneous removal of renal calculi. RadioGraphics 1985;5: 149-69.

Cragg A, Lund G, Rysavy J, Castaneda F, Castaneda-Zuniga WR, Amplatz K. Nonsurgical placement of arterial endoprostheses: a new technique using Nitinol wire. Radiology 1983;147:261-3.

Cramer R, Moore R, Amplatz K. Reduction of the surgical complication rate by the use of a hypothrombogenic catheter coating. Radiology 1973;109:585-8.

Epstein DH, Darcy MD, Hunter DW, Coleman CC, Tadavarthy SM, Murray PD et al. Experience with the Amplatz retrievable vena cava filter. Radiology 1989; 172:105-10.

Fernström I, Johansson B. Percutaneous pyelolithotomy: a new extraction technique. Scand J Urol Nephrol 1976;10:257-9.

Frech RS, Cramer R, Amplatz K. A simple noninvasive technique to test nonthrombogenic surfaces. Am J Roentgen Radium Ther Nucl Med 1971;113:765-8.

Goodwin WE, Casey WC, Woolf W. Percutaneous trocar (needle) nephrostomy in hydronephrosis. JAMA 1955;157:891-4.

Herrera M, Rysavy J, Kotula F, Rusnak B, Castaneda-Zuniga WR, Amplatz K. Ivalon shavings: technical considerations of a new embolic agent. Radiology 1982;144:638-40.

Lagrave G, Plessis JK, Pougeard-Dulimbert G, Passicos J. Lithiase biliary residuelle; extraction a la sonde Dormia par le drain de Kehr. Mem Acad Chir (Paris) 1969;14:431-5.

Leslie J, Amplatz K, Korbuly D, Waltz F. A new simple power injector. Am J Roentgen 1977;128:381-4.

Lund G, Rysavy J, Hunter DW, Castaneda-Zuniga WR, Amplatz K. Retrievable vena caval filter percutaneously introduced. Radiology 1985;155:831.

Lund G, Rysavy JA, Salomonowitz E, Cragg AH, Kotula F, Casteneda-Zuniga WR et al. A new vena caval filter for percutaneous placement and retrieval: experimental study. Radiology 1984;152:369-72.

Pfister RC, Newhouse JH. Interventional percutaneous pyeloureteral technicques II. Radiol Clin North Am 1979;17:351-63.

Robinson JD, Hunter DW, Castaneda-Zuniga WR, Amplatz K. A new torque guide wire. Radiology 1987;165:572-3.

Rusnak B, Castaneda-Zuniga, Kotula F, Herrera M, Amplatz K. An improved dilator system for percutaneous nephrostomies. Radiology 1982;144:174.

Seldinger SI. Catheter replacement of the needle in percutaneous arteriography; new technique. Acta Radiol 1953;39:368-76.

Smith AD, Reinke DB, Miller RP, Lange PH. Percutaneous nephrostomy in the management of ureteral and renal calculi. Radiology 1979;133:49-54.

Smith AD, Lange PH, Fraley EE. Applications of percutaneous nephrostomy. New challenges and opportunities in endo-urology [letter]. J Urol 1979; 121:382.

Smith TP, Darcy MD, Hunter DW, Castaneda-Zuniga WR, Amplatz K. New super-stiff guide wire. Radiology 1986;161:551-2.

Smith TP, Darcy MD, Hunter DW, Castaneda-Zuniga WR, Amplatz K. A new retention catheter. Radiology 1986;160:559-60.

Smith TP, Derauf BJ, Darcy MD, Hunter DW, Castaneda-Zuniga WR, Amplatz K. Movable core guide wire: evaluation of improved model. Radiology 1986;159:552-3.

Stables DP, Ginsberg NJ, Johnson ML. Percutaneous nephrostomy: a series and review of the literature. Am J Roentgen 1978;130:75-82.

Tadarvarthy SM, Knight L, Ovitt TW, Snyder C, Amplatz, K. Therapeutic transcatheter arterial embolization. Radiology 1974;112:13-6.

Tadarvarthy SM, Coleman C, Hunter D, Casteneda-Zuniga WR, Amplatz K. Dual stiffness Malecot (Stamey) catheter. Radiology 1984;152:225.

Wallace S, Gianturco C, Anderson JH, Goldstein HM, Davis LJ, Bree RL. Therapeutic vascular occlusion utilizing steel coil technique: clinical applications. Am J Roentgen 1976;127:381-7.

Wickbom I. Pyelography after direct puncture of the renal pelvis. Acta Radiol 1954;41:505-12.

Zollikofer C, Castaneda-Zuniga WR, Galliani C, Rysavy JA, Formanek A, Amplatz K. Therapeutic blockade of arteries using compressed Ivalon. Radiology 1980;136:635-40.

Zollikofer CL, Salomonowitz E, Sibley R, Chain J, Bruehlmann WF, Castaneda-Zuniga WR et al. Transluminal angioplasty evaluated by electron microscopy. Radiology 1984;153:369-74.

Chapter 9

Anderson JH, Wallace S, Gianturco C. Transcatheter intravascular coil occlusion of experimental arteriovenous fistulas. Am J Roentgen 1977;129:795-8.

Anderson JH, Wallace S, Gianturco C, Gerson LP. "Mini" Gianturco stainless steel coils for transcatheter vascular occlusion. Radiology 1979;132:301-3.

Camp JD, Gianturco C. A simplified technique for roentgenographic examination of the optic canals. Am J Roentgen Radium Ther 1933;29:547-9.

Carrasco CH, Wallace S, Charnsangavej C, Richli W, Wright KC, Fanning T et al. Expandable biliary endoprosthesis: an experimental study. Am J Roentgen 1985;145:1279-81.

Charnsangavej C, Wallace S, Wright KC, Carrasco CH, Gianturco C. Endovascular stent for use in aortic dissection: an in vitro experiment. Radiology 1985;157:323-4.

Charnsangavej C, Carrasco CH, Wallace S, Wright KC, Ogawa K, Richli W et al. Stenosis of the vena cava: preliminary assessment of treatment with expandable metallic stents. Radiology 1986;161:295-8.

Chuang VP, Wallace S, Gianturco C. A new improved coil for tapered-tip catheter for arterial occlusion. Radiology 1980;135:507-9.

Cragg A, Lund G, Rysavy J, Castaneda F, Castaneda-Zuniga WR, Amplatz K. Nonsurgical placement of arterial endoprostheses: a new technique using nitinol wire. Radiology 1983;147:261-3.

Desjardins AU, Counseller VS, Gianturco C. Results of treatment in tumors of the testis. Am J Surg 1935; 27:71-8.

Dotter CT. Transluminally placed coilspring endarterial tube grafts. Invest Radiol 1969;4:329-32.

Dotter CT, Buschmann RW, McKinney MK, Rösch J. Transluminal expandable nitinol coil stent grafting: preliminary report. Radiology 1983;147:259-60.

Duprat G, Wright KC, Charnsangavej C, Wallace S, Gianturco C. Flexible balloon-expanded stent for small vessels. Radiology 1987;162:276-8.

Duprat G, Wright K, Charnsangavej C, Wallace S, Gianturco C. Self-expanding metallic stents for small vessels: an experimental evaluation. Radiology 1987;162:469-72.

Gianturco C, Alvarez WC. Roentgen ray motion pictures of the stomach. Proc Staff Meet Mayo Clin 1932;7:669-71.

Gianturco C. Some mechanical factors of gastric physiology. Study I: The empty stomach and various ways of filling. Am J Roentgen Radium Ther 1934; 31:735-44.

Gianturco C. Some mechanical factors of gastric physiology. Study II: The pyloric mechanism. Am J Roentgen Radium Ther 1934;31:745-50.

Gianturco C, Anderson JH, Wallace S. Mechanical devices for arterial occlusion. Am J Roentgen Radium Ther Nucl Med 1975;124:428-35.

Gianturco C, Anderson JH, Wallace S. A new vena cava filter: experimental animal evaluation. Radiology 1980;135:835-7.

Gunther RW, Schild H, Fries A, Storkel S. Vena caval filter to prevent pulmonary embolism: experimental study. Radiology 1985;156:315-20.

Katsamouris AA, Waltman AC, Delichatsios MA, Athanasoulis CA. Inferior vena cava filters: in vitro comparison of clot trapping and flow dynamics. Radiology 1988;166:361-6.

Leddy ET, Gianturco C. The analgesic effect of roentgen rays in metastasis from carcinoma of the prostate gland. Am J Roentgen Radium Ther 1933;29:667-70.

Lund G, Rysavy JA, Salomonowitz E, Cragg AH, Kotula F, Casteneda-Zuniga WR et al. A new vena caval filter for percutaneous placement and retrieval: experimental study. Radiology 1984;152:369-72.

Novy SB, Wallace S, Goldman AM, Ben-Menacham Y. Pyogenic Liver Abscess (Angiographic Diagnosis and Treatment by Closed Aspiration). Am J Roentgen Radium Ther Nucl Med 1974;121:388-395.

Roehm JOF, Gianturco C, Barth MH, Wright KC. Percutaneous transcatheter filter for the inferior vena cava. Radiology 1984;150:255-7.

Roehm JOF, Johnsrude IS, Barth MH, Gianturco C. The bird's nest inferior vena cava filter: progress report. Radiology 1988;168:745-9.

Rollins N, Wright KC, Charnsangavej C, Wallace S, Gianturco C. Self-expanding metallic stents: preliminary evaluation in an atherosclerotic model. Radiology 1987;163:739-42.

Uchida BT, Putnam JS, Rösch J. Modifications of Gianturco expandable wire stents. Am J Roentgen 1988;150:1185-7.

Wallace MJ, Charnsangavej C, Ogawa K, Carrasco CH, Wright KC, McKenna R et al. Tracheobronchial tree: expandable metallic stents used in experimental and clinical applications. Radiology 1986;158:309-12.

Wallace S, Gianturco C, Anderson JH, Goldstein HM, Davis LJ, Bree RL. Therapeutic vascular occlusion utilizing steel coil technique: clinical applications. Am J Roentgen 1976;127:381-387.

Wright KC, Wallace S, Charnsangavej C, Carrasco CH, Gianturco C. Percutaneous endovascular stents: an experimental evaluation. Radiology 1985;156:69-72.

Yune HY. Inferior vena cava filter: search for an ideal device. Radiology 1989;172:15-6.

Chapter 10

Dodd GD, Greening RR, Wallace S. In: Nealon TF. Management of the patient with cancer. Philadelphia: WB Saunders Co., 1965:72-112.

Fraimw W, Wallace S, Greening RR, Cathcart RT. Pulmonary function studies. Cancer Chemother Reports 1968;52:99-105.

Hamilton W, Riley RL, Attyah AM, et al. Comparison of the Fick and dye injection methods of measuring the cardiac output in man. Am J Physiol 1948;153:309-21.

Hudack SS, McMaster PD. Lymphatic participation in human cutaneous phenomena; study of minute lymphatics of living skin. J Exper Med 1933;57:751-74.

Jackson L, Wallace S, Schaeffer B, Gould J, Kramer S, Weiss AJ. The diagnostic value of lymphangiography. Ann Intern Med 1961;54:870-82.

Kato T, Nemoto R, Mori H et al. Arterial chemoembolization with Mitomycin C microcapsules in the treatment of primary or secondary carcinoma of the kidney, liver, bone and interpelvic organs. Cancer 1981;48:674-80.

Kinmouth JB. Lymphangiography in man. Method of outlining lymphatic trunks at operation. Clin Sc 1952;11:13-20.

Nealon T. The Management of the Patient with Cancer. Vol III. Philadelphia: WB Sanders Co, 1965.

Wallace S, Jackson L, Schaffer R, Gould J, Greening RR, Weiss A et al. Lymphangiograms: their diagnostic and therapeutic potential. Radiology 1961;76:179-99.

Wallace S, Jackson L. Diagnostic criteria for lymphagiographic interpretation of malignant neoplasia. Cancer Chemother Reports 1968;52:125-45.

Wallace S, Jing BS, Zornosa J, Hammond JA, Hamberger A, Herson J. Is lymphangiography worthwhile? Int J Radiat Oncol Biol Phys 1979;5:1873-6.

Wallace S, Jing BS, Zornoza J. Lymphangiography in the determination of the extent of metastatic carcinoma. Cancer 1977;39:706-18.

Wright KC, Wallace S, Mosier B, Mosier D. Microcapsules for arterial chemoembolization: appearance and in vitro drug release characteristics. J Microencapsul 1988;5:13-20.

Yang DJ, Wallace S, Tansey W, Wright KC, Kuang LR, Tilbury RS et al. Synthesis and in vitro receptor binding studies of fluorotamoxifen analogues. Pharm Res 1991;8:174-7.

Chapter 11

Cope C. Simple method for the introduction of large-gauge plastic catheters. N Engl J Med 1958;258:1000-2.

Cope C. New pleural biopsy needle: preliminary study. JAMA 1958;167:1107-8.

Cope C. Technique for transseptal catheterization of the left atrium: preliminary report. J Thorac Surg 1959;37:482-6.

Cope C. A new maneuverable guide for selective abdominal catheterization. J Appl Physiol 1961;16:917-8.

Cope C. Useful modification of the Cournand needle. Am Rev Respir Dis 1962;86:936.

Cope C, Bernhardt H. Hook-needle biopsy of pleura, pericardium, peritoneum and synovium. Am J Med 1963;35:189-95.

Cope C. Selective bronchial catheterization by a new percutaneous transtracheal technique. Am J Roentgen Radium Ther Nucl Med 1966;96:932-5.

Cope C. A new safety device for retrograde power femoral aortography. Radiology 1967;88:797-8.

Cope C. A new one-catheter torque-guide system for percutaneous exploratory abdominal angiography. Radiology 1969;92:174-5.

Cope C. Improved anchoring of nephrostomy catheters: loop technique. Am J Roentgen 1980;135:402-3.

Cope C. Use of crossed-limb loop anchor for percutaneous biliary bypass. Am J Roentgen 1982;138:974-6.

Cope C. Replacement of obstructed loop and pigtail nephrostomy and biliary drains. Am J Roentgen 1982;139:1022-3.

Cope C. Stiff fine-needle guide wire for catheterization and drainage. Radiology 1983;147:264.

Cope C. Improved fine needle catheter introducing set for safer central vein cannulation. J Parenter Enteral Nutr 1984;8:594-5.

Cope C. Suture anchor for visceral drainage. Am J Roentgen 1986;146:160-2.

Cope C, Burke DR, Meranze SG. Atlas of Interventional Radiology. New York: Gower Pub, 1990.

Cope C. Conversion from small (0.018 inch) to large (0.038) guide wires in percutaneous drainage procedures. Am J Roentgen 1982;138:170-1.

Index

A

Abele, John 64, 67-68
Abrams, Herbert L 35, 47-48, 66, 128
Adams, DF 48
Albert Einstein Medical Center 121
Almen, T 20
Alvarez, Walter C 91, 99
American Cystoscope Makers Incorporated 14
Amplatz, Kurt 17, 79-89, 126, 128-133
Amplatz portable CO_2-powered injector 80
Anderson, James H 92-93
Andreas Gruentzig Cardiovascular Center 77
angiocardiography 50, 58, 64-65
angioplasty 43, 53-54, 56-57, 67-68, 71-72, 74-77, 83, 87-89, 96-98, 101, 128, 131, 109
arterial embolization 93, 101, 105, 110
arterial plugs 101

B

balloon catheter 13, 14, 33, 57, 58, 59-60, 69, 73-76, 83, 91, 95-96, 101, 115, 122, 124-127, 130, 131
Bartley, O 84, 129
Baum, S 47
Becton-Dickinson 12, 114-115, 125
Belknap, HD 14, 124
Benique, M 13, 122
benzalkonium-heparin coating 82
Berberich, J 20, 123
Bierman, HR 24, 27
Bilbao, MK 63, 65
Bildsoe, Mark C 82, 133
biliary stent set 79
biopsy device 114, 127
Bird's Nest filter 91, 94-95, 108
Boijsen, Erik 31-35, 49-50, 110, 127, 129
Brooks, B 20, 123
Bruun, S 103
Burke, DR 120
Butto, F 83

C

Camp, John D 91
Cardella, JF 83, 86
cardiac catheterization 41, 88
Carle Clinic 91-92, 99-100, 108
Castaneda, F 87
Castaneda-Zuniga, Wilfrido R 85, 87
Charles Dotter Institute of Interventional Therapy 69
chemoembolization 103, 105-107, 111
Cleveland Clinic 37-38, 41, 49, 73
coils, embolizing 91-94, 99-100, 105, 108-109, 131
coils, stent 86
coils, wire guide 17, 83, 129
Coleman, CC 85, 89
contrast medium 16, 20, 24-27, 31-33, 37-39, 41, 45, 48-49, 58, 60, 71, 75, 80-81, 84-85, 88, 97, 116, 123, 127
Cook Incorporated 11, 17-19, 47, 54-55, 62, 66-67, 69, 76, 88, 92, 100, 110, 121, 128-129, 135
Cook Group Incorporated 69, 135
Cook, William A 17, 46, 54-55, 60, 66-69, 73, 75, 92, 101, 135
Cope, Constantin 113-121, 125, 127-130, 132
Cope Gastrointestinal Suture Set 119
Cope Guidewire Exchange System 120
Cope hooked biopsy needle 114
Cordis Corporation 16-17, 19, 46-47, 50, 127-128
Cornell University Medical School 64
coronary angiography 20, 26, 37-38, 41, 43, 45-46, 48-50, 57, 71, 88, 125
coronary angioplasty 71-72, 75-77, 131
Cournand, Andre 15-16, 115, 125-126
Cournand needle 115
Cragg, AH 86, 132
Cramer, Ralph 82, 130
crossed-limb loop (CLL) catheter 117-118

D

Dechamps aneurysm needle 15
Desilets, Donald 17
Desilets-Hoffman catheter introducers 17

Dodd, GD 104, 108, 128
Donald, D 17, 24-25, 126
Dormia basket 85, 130
Dotter, Charles T 9, 13, 17-18, 20, 23, 29, 32, 47, 49-50, 53-69, 71, 73-74, 86-87, 95, 101, 125-132
Dotter dilatation set 55
dottering 54-55, 57, 73, 129
drainage 14, 79, 82, 84-86, 98, 104, 113, 117-121, 124, 126, 128-129, 131-132
Duke University 64
Dunn Foundation for Immunologic Sciences 100, 110
Dunn, John S, Sr 92, 110
Duprat, G 97-98

E

East Orange Veterans Administration Hospital 121
Eastman Kodak 19, 123
Edholm, P 27, 126
Eidgenossischen Technischen Hochschule 74
embolization 34, 58, 63, 72, 83, 92-93, 99-101, 103, 105-106, 110-111, 130-131
Emory University 73, 76-77
endourology 84, 88
Engeset, A 103
English scale 14
Espy, Larry 87
exit catheterization 61-62, 130

F

Fariñas, PL 24-25
Federal University of LaPlata 42
Fell, EH 65
Fernström, I 84-85
film changer 66, 81
Foley, Frederic EB 14, 117, 124
Forestier, G 20, 123
Forssmann, Werner 9, 15
Fraser, DB 48
Frech, Robert S 82
French (F) scale 14, 123
Frische, Lou H 57

G

Ganz, William   57, 59, 130
Gelfoam   83, 93, 105-106
Gerow, JW   14, 124
Gershon-Cohen, Jacob   121
Gianturco, Cesare   55, 73, 91-101, 108-109, 124-125, 131-133
Gianturco-Roubin Flex Stent Coronary Stent   101
Gidlund, A   31, 127
Goodwin, Willard E   84, 126
Greening, RR   104, 128
Gruentzig, Andreas   55, 71-77, 96, 101, 130-131

H

Haschek, F   20, 123
Heidelberg Medical School   75
Henry Ford Hospital   41
heparin coating   17, 81-82, 88
Hirsch, S   20, 123
Hoffman, Richard   17
Holland   103
Horvath, Laszlo   65
Hreshchyshyn, MM   103
Hudack, SS   103
Hurst, JW   72, 76

I

interventional radiology   1, 9, 21, 26, 28, 34, 55, 59, 74, 88, 100, 103, 108, 110-111, 113, 120-121
Ivalon   83, 106, 131

J

Jayne, Zophar   10
Jeckel, Norman   16
Jefferson Medical College   103, 110
Jefferson University Hospital   100
Jennings, Ross   11, 67
Johns Hopkins   38
Jönsson, Gunnar   20, 24
Judkins, Melvin P   17, 23, 32-33, 35, 41, 45-51, 57, 62, 68, 73, 87, 128-129

K

Karolinska Institute   16, 28
Kato, T   106
Katsamouris, AA   95
Kennedy Veterans Administration Hospital   121
Kidd, Harold J   68
KIFA   16, 18, 127
King's County Hospital   120
King, Spencer   77
Kinmouth, JB   103
Kirklin, BR   91
Kotula, Frank   87
Kuder, K   65

L

Leddy, ET   91
Ledin   16, 127
Lewis, Royston   39
Lindenthal, OT   20, 123
liver-biopsy catheter   61
locking collar   60
Loma Linda University   49-50
loop-snare catheter   63
Lower Bucks County Hospital   110
Lower, Richard   15
lymph-node biopsies   104
lymphangiography   100, 103-104, 108, 128

M

MD Anderson Hospital and Tumor Institute   92, 100, 104, 109, 110
Machlett Laboratories   56
Major, Johann Daniel   10
Malecot   79, 84, 88, 117, 132
Malecot abscess-drainage set   79
Malecot nephrostomy drainage catheter   117
Malek, P   103
Malmö General Hospital   33
Markowitz   105
Max Rataschow Hospital   75
Mayo Clinic   18, 49, 88, 91, 99
McMaster, PD   103
mechanical dissolution of clots   82, 133
Medi-Tech   19, 67-68, 129
Meranze, SG   120
Mercier, LA   13
metastatic neuroendocrine tumors   106
microencapsulation   106-107
Moniz, E   20
Morgan, Russell   38
Mosier, Benjamin   106
Muller Tip Deflecting System   19, 127

N

National Cash Register Company   106
National Institutes of Health   56, 68, 134
Nealon, T   104
needle-biopsy instrument   114
Nelaton, Auguste   13
New York Medical College   120
nitinol   64, 86, 132
Nordenstrom, B   32
Neuner, A   10
Nuvoli, I   20, 124

O

Ödman, Per   16, 31
Olin, Tord   31, 32, 49
Olsson, Olle   31, 49
Oregon Health Sciences University   69
Osborne, Tom   18, 92, 100

P

Peirce, EC   24-25
percutaneous entry   9, 12, 16-17, 24, 26, 28, 31-32, 41, 45, 64, 83-84, 126
percutaneous transluminal angioplasty (PTA)   53-54, 128
percutaneous transluminal coronary angioplasty (PTCA)   71, 76, 131
Philadelphia General Hospital   110
Phillips Company   38
pigtail catheter   33, 48, 50, 129
Porstmann, Werner   17, 57, 60, 65, 73, 101, 129, 131
Pravaz, Charles-Gabriel   11
Prokopek   103

R

Racine, Maurice   20, 124
Radner, S   24, 125
Rappaport, AM   24, 27, 126
Reybard, Jean François   13, 122
Reyboul, Henri   20, 124
Ricketts, HJ   47, 128

Rigler, Leo 88
Robb-Steinberg angiocardiography needle 58
Robinson, JD 83
Rodriguez-Alvarez, A 31, 127
Roehm, John OF, Jr 95
Roentgen, Wilhelm Conrad 9, 19-20
Rollins, Nancy 97
Rösch, Josef 109
Roswell Park Hospital 103
Roto-Flector tip-straightening system 19, 127
Roubin, G 96
Ruble, Enid 66
Rusnak, B 85, 132
Ruttenberg, Herbert 17

S

Safe-T-J wire guide 17, 47, 62, 69, 129
Schick X-Ray 18
Schlumpf, Maria 74, 76
Schlumpf, Walter 74
Schneider Company 75
Schneider, Karl 12
Scottish scale 14
Seldinger, Sven I 9, 16, 18, 23-29, 31-32, 35, 41, 45, 64-65, 72, 83, 116, 125-126
Seldinger percutaneous entry technique 23, 25-26, 31-32, 35, 45, 65, 83, 116
septal defect occluder 101
Servelle, M 103
Sheehan, FR 103
Sheridan, David 16
Sicard, JA 20, 123
Simonsgaard, Christian 97
Smith, AD 83-85
Sones, Mason, Jr 26, 37-43, 45-46, 48-50, 126-127, 131
Sones technique 26, 41-42, 45
squirt catheter 60, 130
St. Johns Hospital 88
Stables, DP 84
Stanford University 33
Starr, Albert 49
steerable catheter system 116, 130
Steinberg, Israel 64
stents 76, 83-84, 86, 91, 95-100, 108-110, 133

Stevens, Robert C 16-17, 46, 48, 50, 128
Straube, Kurt R 58
Strax, Philip 68
Stueve, Richard 50
Sussman, ML 65
Swan, HJC 57, 59, 130
Swan-Ganz catheter 59

T

Tadavarthy, SM 83-84, 131-132
Temple University 110
Temple University School of Medicine 121
Thomas Jefferson University 103, 110
Thompson, Sir Henry 14
thromboresistant coatings 81
Tillander, H 25, 27, 125
Tornvall, G 32
transhepatic cholangiography 28, 104
transluminal angioplasty 53, 56-57, 67, 75, 87, 89, 128
transseptal technique 114-115, 127
transtracheal catheterization 116, 129

U

US Naval Hospital 64
Uchida, Barry T 96, 98
United States Catheter and Instrument Corporation (USCI) 16-17, 19, 38-41, 125, 127-128, 131
University Hospital (Lund and Helsingborg) 33
University Hospital (Zurich) 73
University Hospital Polyclinic 75
University of Berlin 15, 99
University of California at Los Angeles 17
University of Illinois 100
University of Innsbruck 88
University of London 75, 120
University of Lund 31, 33, 35, 49
University of Maryland 41-42
University of Minnesota 79, 84-85, 87-88, 99
University of Naples 99
University of Oregon 49-50, 54, 64, 67-68
University of Oregon Hospital 54
University of Pennsylvania, Hospital of 121
University of Rome 99
University of Zurich 76
ureteral stent set 79, 88

V

vascular catheters 14-17, 122
vascular obstruction set 79
vena cava filter 86, 94-95, 101, 132
Veterinary School (Lyon, France) 11

W

Wallace, Sidney 26, 35, 92-93, 98, 103-112, 128, 130-131, 133
Wayne State University 88
West Haven Veterans Administration Hospital 121
Western Maryland College 41-42
Wickbom, I 83, 126
William Cook Europe 60, 73, 75
wire guide 9, 17-18, 23-25, 32, 46-47, 53-56, 59, 62-63, 65, 69, 79, 82-86, 88, 125-128, 129-130, 132, 135
Wirtanen, GW 105
Witting, Vito 99
Wood, Alexander 10-11
Wren, Christopher 10
Wright, KC 96, 99, 133
Wulfing-Lüer 12
Würzburg 19

Y

Yang, David 107

Z

zigzag (Z) stents 95-98, 109, 133
Zollikofer, C 83, 87